Contents

Introduction
Coronavirus and diabetes

****

AN EMERALD GUIDE

TO

EXPLAINING DIABETES

DOREEN JARRETT

Editor: Roger Sproston

533 783 15 3

Emerald Guides

© Straightforward C o Ltd 2022

ISBN

978-1-80236-092-9

Printed by 4edge www.4edge.co.uk

Cover design by BW Studio Derby

Introduction

You may be reading this book (Revised Edition 2022) because you have either contracted diabetes and want to know more or one of your loved ones or friends has the condition, or you are just generally interested. Either way, diabetes is more and more prevalent now than ever before and it is necessary for everyone affected, or potentially affected, to have a knowledge of the condition, how it arises, what are the implications and symptoms and how to control it.

There are certain common factors associated with diabetes: type 1 diabetes is treated with insulin and type 2 with a general range of tablet-based medications. However, one very important factor here is the lifestyle of the diabetic. Of equal importance alongside diet and medication is diet and exercise.

This book is an introduction to diabetes and seeks to explain the nature of the condition, the symptoms, how to control the symptoms and how to adjust one's lifestyle to ensure that the effects of diabetes are minimised and, in some cases, eradicated altogether. Chapter 1 begins by explaining diabetes. chapter 2 discusses symptoms, chapter 3 diabetes care, chapter 4 diet and exercise, chapter 5 medications used in diabetes and chapter 6 advances in diabetes care.

How coronavirus can affect people with diabetes

The majority of people who do get Coronavirus – whether they have diabetes or not – will have mild symptoms and don't need to go into hospital. However, everyone with diabetes, including those with type 1, type 2, gestational and other types, is more vulnerable to developing a severe illness if they do get coronavirus.

In adults with diabetes, there are certain factors that increase risk of serious illness like being older, having a high HbA1c, or having a history of diabetes-related complications. There are other factors too, like your BMI and ethnicity, that research shows can have an impact on your risk. In children with diabetes, the risk of becoming seriously ill with coronavirus is very low.

Being ill can make your blood sugar go all over the place. Your body tries to fight the illness by releasing stored glucose (sugar) into your blood stream to give you energy. But your body can't produce enough or any insulin to cope with this, so your blood sugars rise.

Your body is working overtime to fight the illness, making it harder to manage your diabetes. This means you're more at risk of having serious blood sugar highs and lows, potentially leading to DKA (diabetic ketoacidosis) or HHS (hyperosmolar hyperglycaemic state).

Lateral flow tests

Rapid lateral flow tests are available to encourage people to test themselves regularly. You can buy rapid lateral flow tests from a pharmacy.

Managing your blood glucose (sugar) levels

Research has shown that having a high HbA1c can increase your risk of becoming seriously ill from coronavirus. So it's important to work with your diabetes team to try to bring your blood sugar levels to a healthy range.

Getting the coronavirus vaccine

The most important way people living with diabetes can lower their risk of becoming seriously ill from coronavirus is to avoid catching the virus in the first place. A vaccine is the most effective way to prevent infection. All adults aged 16 and over, including people with diabetes, have now been invited to have their vaccine.

Children aged 12 to 15 are now being offered the Pfizer-BioNTech vaccine. Parents and guardians will get a letter with information about when the vaccine will be offered. Most children will be given their vaccine at school.

Booster vaccines

The booster vaccination programme has been extended for all people aged 18 and over.

Face masks

Wearing a mask helps keep you and others safe and is a simple way to reduce your risk as you go about your daily life.

A legal requirement to wear a face covering in certain settings remains in place in some settings in Scotland, Wales and Northern Ireland:

- In Scotland, masks must be worn in shops, on public transport, at work as well as in pubs, cafes and restaurants when not seated.
- In Wales, masks are legally required on public transport, in taxis and in all public indoor areas apart from pubs and restaurants.
- In Northern Ireland, as of 15/02/2022 face coverings are no longer a legal requirement. It is still strongly recommended in health and social care settings, on public transport and in enclosed indoor settings, where you come into contact with people you do not usually meet however.

If you get coronavirus

If you do get coronavirus, it's really important that you follow your sick day rules. This will help you to keep your blood sugars in range as much as possible, so you can stay well and fight the virus. We know it's not that always that simple. Some people are being treated for coronavirus with a steroid called dexamethasone, which can make your blood sugars go high. Find out more about the steroid dexamethasone and diabetes.

How coronavirus can affect children with diabetes

Children typically have mild symptoms if they catch the virus. However, as with all people with diabetes, an illness like coronavirus can make it harder to manage your child's diabetes and the risk of DKA will be higher when they are unwell. A vaccine is the most effective way to prevent getting ill from coronavirus.

How coronavirus can affect pregnant women with diabetes

The same rules apply to you as for everyone with diabetes. If you're pregnant and have diabetes, then you are not more at risk of getting the virus. However, if you do get the virus, you could be more at risk of developing complications and it could become harder to manage your diabetes. For that reason, it's really important you're extra careful and follow social distancing rules.

You can find all the latest information for pregnant women from the Royal College of Obstetricians and Gynaecologists www.rcog.org.uk

How coronavirus can affect people in type 2 diabetes remission

Diabetes remission works differently for different people, and we still don't know enough about it. So we don't know for sure how the virus could affect you if you're in remission. Everyone, including people in diabetes remission, should carefully follow social distancing rules.

How coronavirus can affect people from Black, Asian and minority ethnic groups

The risk of death from coronavirus for some ethnic groups is higher than for people of white ethnicity. But it is important to remember that there are lots of factors involved, like age, and overall risk of dying from coronavirus is very low.

In England and Wales, data from the Office of National Statistics shows how people from certain Black, Asian and minority ethnic (BAME) groups are more at risk than people of white ethnicity. Research in Scotland hasn't shown this increased risk, but the BAME population there is very small.

Can coronavirus cause diabetes?

There is growing evidence to suggest that coronavirus might be triggering diabetes in some people, or making the condition worse for others. We've taken a look at the research so far and explain what scientists are doing to find answers.

Small studies have suggested that rates of new type 1 diabetes diagnoses in children were higher in 2020 compared to average rates in previous years. The causes of type 1 diabetes are complex, and scientists think that there are a variety of environmental and genetic reasons that could explain why the condition develops. Viruses could be one of these reasons, but the evidence around this is mixed and we just don't know for sure yet.

Advice for clinically extremely vulnerable people

The advice for clinically extremely vulnerable people to 'shield' came to an end in 2021. Shielding was a way of protecting 'clinically extremely vulnerable' people who are at a very high risk of severe illness and needing to go to hospital if they catch coronavirus. It meant staying at home almost all of the time, with no face-to-face contact.

Governments in England, Scotland, Wales and Northern Ireland have each set out their own guidance for people who were listed as clinically extremely vulnerable. Wherever you live, it's still really important to keep following any coronavirus guidance in your area and to shield if you feel it's right for you.

England

The shielding programme has ended in England. This means that people who were previously considered clinically extremely vulnerable (CEV) will not be advised to shield in the future or follow specific national guidance.

Your diabetes team may provide individual advice to you about your risk, depending on your individual situation and any complications or other health conditions you may have. You could raise this at your next routine appointment.

You might also want to continue to take precautions to reduce your risk such as:

- making sure those you are meeting have been vaccinated - you might want to wait until 14 days after everyone's second dose of COVID-19 vaccine before being in close contact with others;
- considering continuing to practice social distancing if that feels right for you and your friends;
- asking friends and family to take a rapid lateral flow antigen test before visiting you;
- asking home visitors to wear face coverings;
- avoiding crowded spaces.

Scotland

There are 5 COVID-19 Protection Levels (0-4) in Scotland. All of Scotland has moved out of the levels system. You can find more information on www.gov.scot/coronavirus

Wales

There are 5 COVID-19 Alert Levels (0-4) in Wales. All of Wales is currently under Alert Level 0. Find out more about these rules on gov.wales/coronavirus

Those who are clinically extremely vulnerable should have got letters with advice on how to stay safe, including things like working from home. After 1 April 2021, the advice for clinically extremely vulnerable people to shield in Wales ended.

Northern Ireland

The advice for people who are clinically extremely vulnerable to shield in Northern Ireland came to an end on 12 April 2021.

If you are clinically extremely vulnerable, the recommendation is to continue to exercise great care and work from home where possible. If it is not possible, you can go to work, provided your employer has taken the proper measures to ensure social distancing.

Find more information on the Northern Ireland government website:

www.nidirect.gov.uk/articles/coronavirus-covid-19-how-stay-safe-and-help-prevent-spread

Going to work

People in England have been told they no longer need to work from home. In Scotland, employers have been asked to consider a 'hybrid' working arrangement from 31 January, where employees spend some time in the office and some time at home. In Wales, from 28 January, the work from home law ended and people are encouraged to work from home if they can. In Northern Ireland, the legal requirement for workplaces to maintain social distancing has ended but people are still encouraged to work from home where possible. Wherever you live in the UK, your employer must make sure your workplace is safe – this means doing a risk assessment at work.

Children and school

Everyone, including children with diabetes, can get coronavirus. The rules about on social distancing and hand washing apply to children with diabetes too.

Schools should be practicing social distancing for your child. This is to prevent the virus from spreading between children and your home. We know this is easier said than done, and can depend on how old your child is and the size of the school.

You may be worried about whether it is safe for your child to go to school if they have diabetes. Speak to the school and to your child's diabetes team about your concerns.

Long COVID

Long COVID is used to describe signs and symptoms that last for a few weeks or months after having a confirmed or suspected case of COVID-19. It can affect your whole body, and your symptoms can change and come and go over time. If you think you might have Long COVID, the first thing you should do is speak to your GP. They will look into your symptoms and first try to find out if there are any other possible causes.

Treatment of Long COVID or COVID fatigue will depend on how long you have been experiencing these symptoms. Treatment is often focused on managing the symptoms and this can vary from person to person.

Your diabetes is unlikely to increase your risk of developing Long COVID. Managing both the symptoms of Long COVID and your diabetes may be difficult but make sure you're aware of your sick day rules and take each day as it comes.

Where can I get more support?

We know some people may not have friends and family able to help while they are staying at home. You may be able to get help from voluntary groups in your area or your local councils or local authorities. Check your government websites for more information. You could also find out if there's a diabetes local group in your area.

Overall, this brief explanation of diabetes should prove invaluable to all who read it.

****

Chapter 1

What is Diabetes?

___

Without a doubt, diabetes (full name Diabetes Mellitus) is one of the most widespread conditions affecting people today, in the United Kingdom and elsewhere. It is one of the oldest known human diseases, and there are several types, one slightly more severe and needing greater control than the other:

- Diabetes 1 (where insulin injections are needed) which most commonly starts in younger patients who need to have regular doses of insulin to stay healthy and:
- Diabetes 2, commonly controlled through the use of tablets, which is usually age related and can be brought on through lifestyle, i.e. lack of exercise and bad diet.

Diabetes is caused through having too much glucose in your blood which results in a change in your internal chemistry. Ultimately, the cause of diabetes is a deficiency of the hormone insulin.

(See overleaf)

Type 1 diabetes

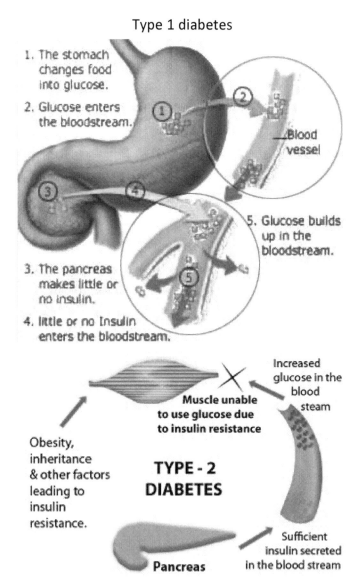

1. The stomach changes food into glucose.

2. Glucose enters the bloodstream.

Blood vessel

5. Glucose builds up in the bloodstream.

3. The pancreas makes little or no insulin.

4. little or no Insulin enters the bloodstream.

Increased glucose in the blood steam

Muscle unable to use glucose due to insulin resistance

Obesity, inheritance & other factors leading to insulin resistance.

TYPE - 2 DIABETES

Sufficient insulin secreted in the blood stream

Pancreas

Who gets diabetes?

Over 4 per cent of people in the UK have diabetes, with many people not realising that they have it. The number is increasing. The vast majority have type 2, and more women than men are affected. This is possibly because diabetes, particularly type 2, occurs later in life and women tend to live longer. However, as the age of the population is rising, type 2 diabetes is likely to become more common as time goes by.

In addition to the UK statistics, the incidence of diabetes is rising worldwide. The numbers of children with type 1 diabetes is on the rise and the numbers of young people with type 2 diabetes is also rising because of the rise in obesity. As the food industry won't really change radically, with fast food just as prevalent, a growing awareness of the damaging effects of food has been promoted. Unfortunately, like a lot of illness, people don't actually sit up and take notice until it happens to them!

Type 1 diabetes and insulin

In the later part of the 19th century, two doctors in Germany discovered the fact that the pancreas-a large gland behind the stomach-produced a substance that regulated the level of blood glucose, stopped it rising. Later in the 20th century scientists isolated this substance and named it insulin. This came from a small group of cells within the pancreas, which were called the Islets of Langerhans.

Insulin became available as a treatment from 1922 onwards and was heralded as a life-saving miracle helping people who otherwise might have died from the condition.

Insulin is a hormone. It works as a chemical messenger that helps your body use the glucose in your blood to give you energy.

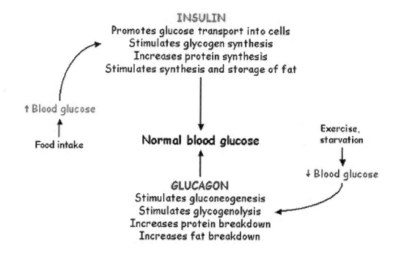

You can think of insulin as the key that unlocks the door to the body's cells. Once the door is unlocked, glucose can enter the cells where it is used as fuel. In Type 1 diabetes the body is unable to produce any insulin so there is no key to unlock the door, and the glucose builds up in the blood.

In essence, what happens is:

- The body can't use glucose to provide energy and tries to get it from elsewhere and starts to break down stores of fat and protein instead. This can cause weight loss. Because the body doesn't use the glucose it ends up passing into the urine. This may be triggered by a virus or other infection.

Type 2 diabetes

Type 2 diabetes usually appears in people over the age of 40, though in South Asian people, who are at greater risk, it often appears from the age of 25. It is also increasingly becoming more common in children, adolescents and young people of all ethnicities. Type 2 diabetes accounts for between 85 and 95 per cent of all people with diabetes and is treated with a healthy diet and increased physical activity. In addition to this, medication and/or insulin are often required, particularly in the early stages.

With type 2 diabetes there is not enough insulin (or the insulin isn't working properly), so the cells are only partially unlocked and glucose builds up in the blood.

Other mechanisms in the body work together with insulin to help maintain the correct levels of glucose, although it is a fact that insulin is the only means that the body has of actually lowering blood glucose levels. After a meal, if there is an insulin deficiency then there will be no brake on the glucose absorbed from what you have eaten and the levels in your blood will carry on rising. When the concentration of glucose rises above a certain level, the glucose will spill out of the bloodstream and into the urine, which can lead to infections.

In addition, excess glucose will lead to the passing of more urine because the glucose in the blood is filtered out by the kidneys, which try to dispose of it by excreting more salt and also water. This is called polyuria and is often the earliest sign of diabetes. If nothing is done to stop or prevent this process dehydration will occur. Insulin also acts to prevent weight loss. Lack of insulin will inevitably lead to weight loss.

There are a number of early indicators of diabetes in a person, the severity of which will depend on the type of diabetes that they have, either type 1 or type 2. The main symptoms are:

- Thirst
- Dehydration
- Passing large quantities of urine
- Infections in the urinary tract, such as cystitis or thrush
- Tiredness and lethargy
- Blurred vision resulting from a dehydrated lens in the eye.

Genetics of Diabetes

Unlike some traits, diabetes does not seem to be inherited in a simple pattern. Yet clearly, some people are born more likely to develop diabetes than others.

What leads to genetic diabetes?

Type 1 and type 2 diabetes have different causes. Yet two factors are important in both. You inherit a predisposition to the disease then something in your environment triggers it.

Genes alone are not enough. One proof of this is identical twins. Identical twins have identical genes. Yet when one twin has type 1 diabetes, the other gets the disease at most only half the time. When one twin has type 2 diabetes, the other's risk is at most 3 in 4.

Type 1 Diabetes

In most cases of type 1 diabetes, people need to inherit risk factors from both parents. Because most people who are at risk do not get diabetes, researchers want to find out what the environmental triggers are.

One trigger might be related to cold weather. Type 1 diabetes develops more often in winter than summer and is more common in places with cold climates. Another trigger might be viruses. Perhaps a virus that has only mild effects on most people triggers type 1 diabetes in others.

Early diet may also play a role. Type 1 diabetes is less common in people who were breastfed and in those who first ate solid foods at later ages.

In many people, the development of type 1 diabetes seems to take many years. In experiments that followed relatives of people with type 1 diabetes, researchers found that most of those who later got diabetes had certain autoantibodies in their blood for years before.

Type 2 Diabetes

Type 2 diabetes has a stronger link to family history and lineage than type 1, although it too depends on environmental factors.

Studies of twins have shown that genetics play a very strong role in the development of type 2 diabetes.

Lifestyle also influences the development of type 2 diabetes. Obesity tends to run in families, and families tend to have similar eating and exercise habits.

If you have a family history of type 2 diabetes, it may be difficult to figure out whether your diabetes is due to lifestyle factors or genetic susceptibility. Most likely it is due to both. However, don't lose heart. Studies show that it is possible to delay or prevent type 2 diabetes by exercising and losing weight. See chapter 4 for an outline of the ideal diet for those with diabetes and also chapter 4 for exercises.

Type 1 Diabetes: Your Child's Risk

In general, if you are a man with type 1 diabetes, the odds of your child developing diabetes are 1 in 17. If you are a woman with type 1 diabetes and your child was born before you were 25, your child's risk is 1 in 25; if your child was born after you turned 25, your child's risk is 1 in 100. Your child's risk is doubled if you developed diabetes before age 11. If both you and your partner have type 1 diabetes, the risk is between 1 in 10 and 1 in 4. There is an exception to these numbers.

About 1 in every 7 people with type 1 diabetes has a condition called type 2 Polyglandular autoimmune syndrome. In addition to having diabetes, these people also have Thyroid disease and a poorly working Adrenal gland. Some also have other Immune system disorders. If you have this syndrome, your child's risk of getting the syndrome — including type 1 diabetes — is 1 in 2.

Tests can also make your child's risk clearer. A special test that tells how the body responds to glucose can tell which School-aged children are most at risk.

Another more expensive test can be done for children who have siblings with type 1 diabetes. This test measures antibodies to insulin, to islet cells in the pancreas, or to an enzyme called glutamic acid decarboxylase. High levels can indicate that a child has a higher risk of developing type 1 diabetes.

Type 2 Diabetes: Your Child's Risk

Type 2 diabetes runs in families. In part, this tendency is due to children learning bad habits-eating a poor diet, not exercising-from their parents. But there is also a genetic basis. In general, if you have type 2 diabetes, the risk of your child getting diabetes is 1 in 7 if you were diagnosed before age 50 and 1 in 13 if you were diagnosed after age 50.

Some scientists believe that a child's risk is greater when the parent with type 2 diabetes is the mother. If both you and your partner have type 2 diabetes, your child's risk is about 1 in 2.

People with certain rare types of type 2 diabetes have different risks. If you have the rare form called maturity-onset diabetes of the young (MODY), your child has almost a 1-in-2 chance of getting it, too.

Maturity onset diabetes of the young (MODY)

MODY is a rare form of diabetes which is different from both Type 1 and Type 2 diabetes, and runs strongly in families. It is caused by a mutation (or change) in a single gene. If a parent has this gene mutation, any child they have has a 50% chance of inheriting it from them. If a child does inherit the mutation they will generally go on to develop MODY before they're 25, whatever their weight, lifestyle or any other factor.

The main features of MODY are a diagnosis of diabetes under the age of 25, having a parent with diabetes, and with diabetes in two or more generations and not necessarily needing insulin.

Types of MODY

There are a number of common types of MODY that have been identified. They are:

- HNF1-alpha. This gene causes about 70% of cases of MODY. It causes diabetes by lowering the amount of insulin made by the pancreas. Diabetes usually develops in adolescence or early twenties, and people with HNF1-alpha MODY generally don't need to take insulin, they can be treated with small doses of a group of tablets called sulphonylureas (often used in Type 2 diabetes). (see medication in chapter 5)
- HNF4-alpha. This isn't as common as the other forms of MODY. People who have inherited a change in this gene are likely to have had a birth weight of 9lb or more (around 4 kg). They may also have had a low blood sugar at, or soon after, birth which might have needed

treatment. The usual treatment is a sulphonylurea tablet but a person may progress on to needing insulin.

- HNF1-beta. People with this type of MODY can have a variety of problems including renal cysts (cysts of the kidneys), uterine abnormalities and gout as well as diabetes. Often the renal cysts can be detected in the womb before a baby is born. Insulin treatment is usually necessary, as well as following a healthy balanced diet and getting regular physical activity.

- Glucokinase. This gene helps the body to recognise how high the blood glucose level is in the body. When this gene isn't working properly the body allows the level of blood glucose to be higher than it should be. Blood glucose levels in people with glucokinase MODY are typically only slightly higher than normal, generally between 5.5-8mmol/l. You don't generally have symptoms of this type of MODY and so it's often picked up through routine testing (eg during pregnancy). You don't need any treatment for glucokinase MODY.

All types of MODY apart from glucokinase carry a risk of the long-term complications of diabetes so you should follow a healthy balanced diet and keep physically active as this helps to maintain good blood glucose and cholesterol levels which in turn reduce the risk of complications. It's important to know if you've got MODY:

- To make sure you get the right treatment and advice for your type of diabetes (eg stopping insulin).
- As there is a 50% chance of a parent passing on MODY to their child, you can consider and discuss the risk to any children you have/plan to have.
- Genetic testing can be offered to other family members

If you think you might have MODY you should discuss testing with your doctor. Testing for MODY involves:

- Having blood taken for pancreatic antibodies and blood or urine tested for C-peptide (your doctor/hospital can do this).
- Having blood taken for genetic testing. Your doctor/hospital will take the blood from you, but they will send it on to the specialist centre in Exeter for it to be tested, along with details of your diagnosis and treatment

Now read the Main Points from Chapter 1.

****

Main Points from Chapter 1

- Without a doubt, diabetes (full name Diabetes Mellitus) is one of the most widespread conditions affecting people today, in the United Kingdom and elsewhere.

- It is one of the oldest known human diseases, and there are several types, one slightly more severe and needing greater control than the other: Diabetes 1 (where insulin injections are needed) which most commonly starts in younger patients who need to have regular doses of insulin to stay healthy and; Diabetes 2, commonly controlled through the use of tablets, which is usually age related and can be brought on through lifestyle, i.e. lack of exercise and bad diet.

- Diabetes is caused through having too much glucose in your blood which results in a change in your internal chemistry. Ultimately, the cause of diabetes is a deficiency of the hormone insulin.

- Unlike some traits, diabetes does not seem to be inherited in a simple pattern. Yet clearly, some people are born more likely to develop diabetes than others.

- MODY is a rare form of diabetes which is different from both Type 1 and Type 2 diabetes, and runs strongly in families. It is caused by a mutation (or change) in a single gene. If a parent has this gene mutation, any child they have has a 50% chance of inheriting it from them. If a child does inherit the mutation they will generally go on to develop MODY before they're 25, whatever their weight, lifestyle or any other factor.

- The main features of MODY are a diagnosis of diabetes under the age of 25, having a parent with diabetes, and with diabetes in two or more generations and not necessarily needing insulin.

****

Chapter 2

Symptoms and Diagnosis of Diabetes

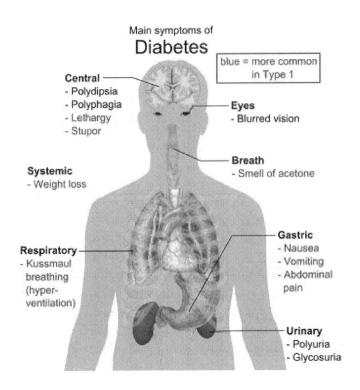

Main symptoms of
Diagnosis of Diabetes

blue = more common
in Type 1

Central
- Polydipsia
- Polyphagia
- Lethargy
- Stupor

Eyes
- Blurred vision

Breath
- Smell of acetone

Systemic
- Weight loss

Gastric
- Nausea
- Vomiting
- Abdominal
  pain

Respiratory
- Kussmaul
  breathing
  (hyper-
  ventilation)

Urinary
- Polyuria
- Glycosuria

As we have seen in the previous chapter, unless you are born with the condition, usually diabetes 1, you can become aware that you have diabetes in several different ways.

The most common symptoms are: (see overleaf)

- Excessive thirst
- Increased urination (sometimes as often as every hour)
- Unexpected weight loss
- Fatigue or tiredness
- Nausea, perhaps vomiting
- Blurred vision
- In women, frequent vaginal infections
- In men and women, yeast infections (thrush)
- Dry mouth
- Slow-healing sores or cuts
- Itching skin, especially in the groin or vaginal area.

Symptoms of type 1 diabetes can develop quickly, over weeks or sometimes days.

Common symptoms of type 2 diabetes

Type 2 diabetes often doesn't cause symptoms and is identified on routine screening. When type 2 diabetes does cause symptoms these can include:

- Excessive thirst
- Increased urination (sometimes as often as every hour), especially at night
- Unexpected weight loss or gain
- Fatigue or extreme tiredness

- Blurred vision
- In women, frequent vaginal infections
- In men and women, yeast infections (thrush)
- Dry mouth
- Slow-healing sores or cuts
- Itching skin, especially in the groin or vaginal area.

Acanthosis nigricans

This is a condition that results in the darkening and thickening of certain areas of the skin, especially in the skin folds. The skin becomes light brown or brown and is sometimes slightly raised and described as velvety. Most often the condition, which typically looks like a small wart, appears on the sides or back of the neck, the armpits, under the breast, and groin. Occasionally the top of the knuckles will have a particularly unusual appearance.

Acanthosis nigricans usually affects people who are very overweight. There is no cure for acanthosis nigricans, but losing weight may improve the condition. Acanthosis nigricans usually precedes diabetes. There are other conditions that are also known to cause acanthosis nigricans, including acromegaly and Cushing Syndrome. Acanthosis nigricans is a skin manifestation of insulin resistance in most people.

Gestational diabetes-See overleaf.

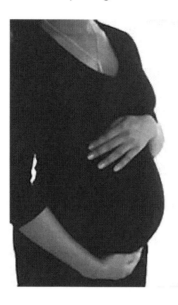

Gestational diabetes is a condition characterised by high blood sugar (glucose) levels that is first recognised during pregnancy. The condition occurs in approximately 14% of all pregnant women.

It is usually diagnosed during routine screening before it causes any symptoms. Seek medical advice about diabetes if:

- You feel nauseated, weak and excessively thirsty; are urinating very frequently; have abdominal pain; or are breathing more deeply and rapidly than normal - perhaps with sweet breath that smells like nail polish remover. You may need immediate medical attention for ketoacidosis, a potentially deadly complication of type 1 diabetes.

- You are having weakness or fainting spells; are experiencing a rapid heartbeat, trembling and excessive sweating; and feel irritable, hungry or suddenly drowsy. You could be developing Hypoglycaemia - low blood sugar that can occur with diabetes treatment. You may need to have a carbohydrate snack or sugary drink promptly to avoid more serious complications.

If you suffer any of the above then the first stop is your GP. Sadly, because of the fact that diabetes is on the rise, your doctor will be only too familiar with the condition and what to do next. The usual step is to take a blood test to measure glucose levels and also take a urine sample. These samples will be sent off to the laboratory, although many doctors surgeries will have blood glucose meters on hand. Some pharmacies also offer blood tests for people who think they may have diabetes.

If you are diagnosed with diabetes then, if it is type 2, your GP will put together a programme of care. If it is type 1 then you would usually be referred to hospital. Following tests the doctor will usually prescribe medicines as outlined in chapter 5.

Problems with eyesight

Diabetic retinopathy is the most common form of eye problem affecting people with diabetes, but further diabetes-related eye problems are common - such as glaucoma and cataracts. Both glaucoma and cataracts can have a serious effect on vision. Diabetic eye disease is a term that encompasses a range of eye problems. On one end of the scale, each of these conditions can cause loss of vision and even blindness but treatments can help to reduce the risk of this happening.

What is diabetic retinopathy?

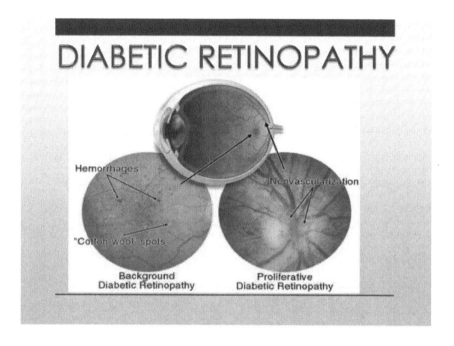

Diabetic retinopathy occurs when changes in blood glucose levels cause changes in retinal blood vessels. In some cases, these vessels will swell up (macular oedema) and leak fluid into the rear of the eye. In other cases, abnormal blood vessels will grow on the surface of the retina. Unless treated, diabetic retinopathy can gradually become more serious and progress from 'background retinopathy' to seriously affecting vision and can lead to blindness. Diabetic retinopathy includes 3 different types:

- Background retinopathy
- Diabetic maculopathy
- Proliferative retinopathy

Symptoms of diabetic retinopathy

Like many conditions of this nature, the early stages of diabetic retinopathy may occur without symptoms and without pain. An actual influence on the vision will not occur until the disease advances.

Macular oedema can result from maculopathy and affect vision occurs if leaking fluid causes the macular to swell. New vessels on the retina can prompt bleeding, which can also block vision in some cases. Symptoms may only become noticeable once the disease advances, but the typical symptoms of retinopathy to look out for include:

- Sudden changes in vision / blurred vision
- Eye floaters and spots
- Double vision
- Eye pain

The longer a person has diabetes, the greater the risk of developing diabetic retinopathy becomes. However, keeping blood glucose levels well controlled can help to significantly slow down the development of retinopathy.

People with diabetes should, however, be aware that a rapid improvement in blood glucose levels can lead to a worsening of retinopathy. A rapid improvement in blood glucose levels in this case is defined as a drop in HbA1c of 30 mmol/mol or 3%.

Preventing diabetic retinopathy

Long-term good blood glucose level management helps to prevent diabetes retinopathy and lower the risk of developing it. Heart disease risk factors also affect retinopathy risk and include stopping smoking, having regular blood pressure and cholesterol checks and undergoing regular eye check-ups.

The risk of developing diabetic retinopathy can be lessened through taking the following precautions:

- Taking a dilated eye examination once a year
- Managing diabetes strictly through medicine, insulin, diet and exercise
- Test blood sugar levels regularly
- Test urine for ketone levels regularly

Treatment of retinopathy

Laser surgery is often used in the treatment of diabetic eye disease, but each stage of diabetic retinopathy can be treated in a different way. Background retinopathy has no treatment but patients will need regular eye examinations.

Maculopathy is usually treated with laser treatment (tiny burns that help to prevent new blood vessel growth and improve the nutrient and oxygen supply to the retina).

Glaucoma and Diabetes

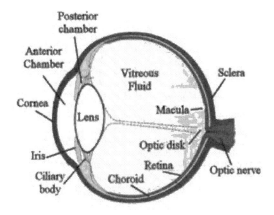

Glaucoma may occur amongst people with and without diabetes, and can be a complication of diabetes if retinopathy develops. Glaucoma is caused by an excess amount of fluid pressing on the nerve at the back of the eye.

How does glaucoma start?

The eye produces a small amount of fluid like water in its middle chamber, which flows around the lens of the eye into the front chamber. The fluid leaves the eye using a drainage network and then enters the bloodstream.

Commonly, glaucoma causes the drainage system to become blocked, and fluid becomes trapped in the eye. This causes pressure to build up in the eye and pass to the nerve at the rear of the eye. This nerve may become damaged by glaucoma.

Is glaucoma linked with diabetes?

People with diabetic retinopathy have an increased risk of glaucoma. This can happen if abnormal blood vessel growth, which can occur as a result of retinopathy, blocks the natural drainage of the eye.

How is glaucoma diagnosed?

Glaucoma may be diagnosed by an optometrist by measuring your eye pressure, checking the eye at the optic nerve, and testing the field of your vision.

A common test these days is a noncontact tonometry test (NCT test) in which a brief puff of air will be directed into the front of your eye. The machine you sit in front of measures the resistance of your eye to the puff of air without needing to make contact with your eye. The puff of air is noticeable but is not painful.

Diabetes and Hypoglycemia

(See overleaf)

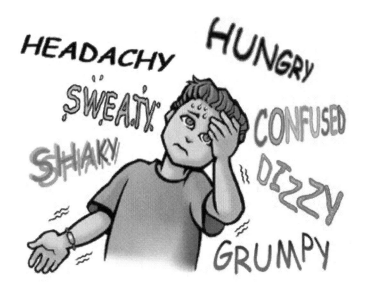

Hypoglycemia (or Hypos) occurs when blood glucose levels fall below 4 mmol/L (72mg/dL). Whilst many people think of diabetes as a problem of high blood sugar levels, the medication some people take can also cause their sugar levels to go too low and this can become dangerous.

Being aware of the early signs of hypoglycemia will allow you to treat your low blood glucose levels quickly - in order to bring them back into the normal range. It is also recommended to make close friends and family aware of the signs of hypoglycemia in case you fail to recognise the symptoms. The main symptoms associated with hypoglycemia are:

- Sweating
- Fatigue
- Feeling dizzy

Other symptoms include:

- Being pale
- Feeling weak
- Feeling hungry
- A higher heart rate than usual
- Blurred vision
- Confusion
- Convulsions
- Loss of consciousness
- And in extreme cases, coma

People affected by hypos

Whilst low blood sugar can happen to anyone, dangerously low blood sugar can occur in people who take the following medication:

- Insulin
- Sulphopnylureas (such as glibenclamide, gliclazide, glipizide, glimepiride, tolbutamide)
- Prandial glucose regulators (such as repaglinide, nateglinide)

Causes of hypoglycemia

Whilst medication is the main factor involved in hypoglycemia within people with diabetes, a number of other factors can increase the risk of hypos occurring. Factors include:

- Too high a dose of medication (insulin or hypo causing tablets)
- Delayed meals
- Exercise
- Alcohol

Diagnosis of hypoglycemia

Hypoglycemia is detected by measuring blood sugar levels with a glucose meter. Any blood glucose level below 4.0 mmol/L indicates that the individual has hypoglycemia. Urine tests do not detect hypoglycemia.

Treating hypoglycemia

A mild case of hypoglycemia can be treated through eating or drinking 15-20g of fast acting carbohydrate such as glucose tablets, sweets, sugary fizzy drinks or fruit juice. Some people with diabetes may also need to take 15-20g of slower acting carbohydrate if the next meal is not due.

A blood test should be taken after 15-20 minutes to check whether blood glucose levels have recovered. Severe hypoglycemia may require an ambulance, for example if loss of consciousness occurs or a seizure persists for more than 5 minutes.

Severe hypos can be treated with glucagon if a glucagon injection kit is available and in date.

Hypoglycemic episodes can range from mild to severe. Mild hypoglycemia can usually be treated by the individual and are to be expected to some degree in people on insulin. Mild hypos are not associated with significant long term health problems unless they are occurring very regularly or for long periods of time.

Severe hypoglycemia, however, will require treatment from someone else and may require an ambulance. Severe hypos can lead to immediate danger if not treated immediately. Whilst rare, severe hypos can potentially lead to coma and death.

Most people experience some warnings before the onset of hypoglycemia. However, some diabetics may experience little or no warning before the onset of sudden or severe hypoglycemia. An impaired ability to spot the signs of hypoglycemia is known as loss of hypo awareness (or hypo unawareness).

Preventing hypoglycemia

The key to preventing hypos is understanding why hypos occur and then taking actions to stop this happening. If you know that a hypo is likely to occur soon, carbohydrates can be taken to raise sugar levels and prevent the hypo. If your doctor is happy for you to adjust your medication doses, you can also lower your dose during or following certain activities (eg exercise or after having alcohol) to prevent a hypo occurring.

Testing blood sugar levels regularly can help you to understand when your sugar levels are dropping too low.

Now read the Main Points from Chapter 2.

****

Main Points from Chapter 2

You can become aware that you have diabetes in several different ways. The most common symptoms are:

- Excessive thirst
- Increased urination (sometimes as often as every hour)
- Unexpected weight loss
- Fatigue or tiredness
- Nausea, perhaps vomiting
- Blurred vision
- In women, frequent vaginal infections
- In men and women, yeast infections (thrush)
- Dry mouth
- Slow-healing sores or cuts
- Itching skin, especially in the groin or vaginal area.

Seek medical advice about diabetes if:

- You feel nauseated, weak and excessively thirsty; are urinating very frequently; have abdominal pain; or are breathing more deeply and rapidly than normal - perhaps with sweet breath that smells like nail polish remover. You may need immediate medical attention for ketoacidosis, a potentially deadly complication of type 1 diabetes.

- You are having weakness or fainting spells; are experiencing a rapid heartbeat, trembling and excessive sweating; and feel irritable, hungry or suddenly drowsy. You could be developing Hypoglycaemia - low blood sugar that can occur with diabetes treatment. You may need to have a carbohydrate snack or sugary drink promptly to avoid more serious complications.

Other problems that can arise from diabetes include :

- Glaucoma
- Eyesight problems (retinopathy)
- Hypoglycemia (Hypos)

****

Chapter 3

General Diabetes Care

Checking glucose levels

As we have outlined in the previous chapters, the point or aim of all treatment for diabetes is to keep the level of glucose in the bloodstream as close as possible to normal.

Monitoring glucose

There are three ways to monitor glucose levels during your initial courses of treatment you will receive advice on the most appropriate way for you. The three methods are as follows:

1. Blood tests for glucose and ketones
2. Continuous subcutaneous glucose monitoring (CGM)
3. Urine tests for glucose and ketones

Blood tests and urine tests are usually taken at a hospital or at your GP surgery.

When your diabetes is being controlled by tablets and/or diet, urine tests are just as effective as blood tests in revealing glucose levels. However, urine tests cannot be used by those who are taking sodium-glucose co-transporter 2 (SGLT2) inhibitors.

Self-blood glucose monitoring

Self-blood glucose monitoring allows you to check your blood glucose levels as often as you need to or as recommended by your doctor.

New guidelines have been produced in March 2022, by the National Institute of Health and Care Excellence (NICE) which recommend wider access to Flash Glucose Monitors and continuous glucose monitoring (CGM) for people living with diabetes on the NHS.

These new guidelines represent a shift towards a better understanding of technology as an integral part of diabetes management, rather than an added luxury.

The new guidelines recommend that:

- all adults with type 1 diabetes should have access to either Flash or CGM
- all children with type 1 diabetes should have access to CGM and that
- some people with type 2 diabetes who use insulin intensive therapy (2 or more injections a day) should have access to Flash, for example if they experience recurrent or severe hypos, if they have a disability that means they cannot finger-prick test or if they would otherwise be advised to test 8 or more times a day.

While NICE only provides recommendations for the NHS in England and Wales, it is hoped that the health service across the UK will adopt these tech recommendations as the minimum standard.

What do I need?

To test blood glucose levels, you need:

- A blood glucose meter
- A lancet device with lancets
- Test strips.

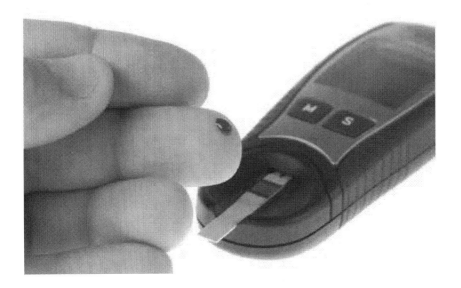

Blood glucose meters are usually sold as kits giving you all the equipment you need to start. There are many different types, offering different features and at different prices to meet individual needs.Your doctor can help you choose the meter that's best for you, and your pharmacist can show you how to use your meter to get accurate results.

How do I test my blood glucose levels?

To test your blood glucose levels, you prick your finger with the lancet and add a small drop of blood onto a testing strip. This strip is then inserted into the meter, which reads the strip and displays a number – your blood glucose level.

When and how often you should test your blood glucose levels varies depending on each individual, the type of diabetes and the tablets and/or insulin being used. Blood glucose levels are measured in millimoles per litre of blood (mmol/L). Your doctor will help you decide how many tests are needed and the levels to aim for.

Keeping a record of your blood glucose levels can be very helpful for you and your doctor You can keep a diary or use a mobile phone app or website to record your levels.

When should I test my blood glucose level?

When you should test your blood glucose levels and how often you should test varies depending on each individual, the type of diabetes and the tablets and/or insulin being used. Your doctor will help you decide how many tests are needed and the levels to aim for. Possible times to test are:

- Before breakfast (fasting)
- Before lunch/dinner
- Two hours after a meal
- Before bed
- Before rigorous exercise
- When you are feeling unwell

Even though your meter may have a memory, it is important to keep a record of your readings in a diary and to take this with you to all appointments with your diabetes health team. This will provide both you and your diabetes health team with important information in deciding if and how your treatment may need to be adjusted.

Most meters on the market have software which allows you to download your records in different formats such as graphs and charts. Even if you can do this, it is still helpful to keep a diary, not only for your tests but also details of your daily activities, the food you eat and other relevant information. There are some apps that record all of this information in one place. Ask your doctor how you can use a diary to help you to better manage your diabetes.

Testing four times a day is usually recommended for people with type 1 diabetes. However many people test more often, such as those using an insulin pump (CSII – continuous subcutaneous insulin infusion).

Why is it so important to test my blood?

Regular testing and recording of your blood glucose level can reinforce your healthy lifestyle choices as well as inform you of your response to other choices and influences.

Importantly, blood glucose level pattern changes can alert you and your health care team to a possible need for a change in how your diabetes is being managed. Testing your blood glucose levels will help you to:

- Develop confidence in looking after your diabetes.
- Better understand the relationship between your blood glucose levels and the exercise you do, the food you eat and other lifestyle influences such as travel, stress and illness.
- Know how your lifestyle choices and medication, if used, are making a difference.
- Find out immediately if your blood glucose levels are too high (hyperglycaemia) or too low (hypoglycaemia), helping you to make important decisions such as eating before exercise, treating a 'hypo' or seeking medical advice if sick.
- Know when to seek the advice of your diabetes nurse about adjusting your insulin, tablets, meal or snack planning when blood glucose goals are not being met.

Times to test more often

There will be times when you need to test more often, Example of these times include when you are:

- Being more physically active or less physically active
- Sick or stressed
- Experiencing changes in routine or eating habits, e.g. travelling
- Changing or adjusting your insulin or medication
- Experiencing symptoms of hyperglycaemia
- Experiencing night sweats or morning headaches
- A female planning pregnancy or are pregnant.
- Pre/post minor surgical day procedures
- Post dental procedures

What should I aim for?

Effective management of diabetes is all about aiming for a careful balance between the foods you eat, how active you are and the medication you take for your diabetes. Because this is a delicate balance, it can be quite difficult to achieve ideal control all the time.

The ranges will vary depending on the individual and an individual's circumstances. While it is important to keep your blood glucose levels as close to the target range of target range between 4 to 6 mmol/L (fasting) as possible to prevent complications,

Glucose level targets

Blood glucose levels are measured in millimoles per litre of blood (mmol/L). Target ranges may differ depending on your age, duration of diabetes, the type of medication you are taking and if you have any other medical problems. Speak with your doctor about your individual target ranges.

Normal blood glucose levels are between 4.0–7.8mmol/L.

Inconsistent highs & lows

Sometimes you may get a lower or higher blood glucose reading than usual and you may not be able to figure out the reason. When you are sick with a virus or flu, your blood glucose levels will nearly always go up and you may need to contact your doctor.

There are a number of other common causes for blood glucose levels to increase or decrease. These include:

- Food – time eaten, type and amount of carbohydrate for example: bread, pasta, cereals, vegetables, fruit and milk
- Exercise or physical activity
- Illness and pain
- Diabetes medication
- Alcohol
- Emotional stress
- Other medications
- Testing techniques.

What if the test result doesn't sound right?

If you're not convinced that a result is correct, here's a suggested check list:

- Have the strips expired?
- Is the strip the right one for the meter?
- Is there enough blood on the strip?
- Has the strip been put into the meter the right way?
- Have the strips been affected by climate, heat or light?
- Did you wash and thoroughly dry your hands before doing the test? (handling sweet foods such as jam or fruit can give higher results)
- Is the meter clean?
- Is the meter too hot or too cold?
- Is the calibration code correct?
- Is the battery low or flat?

All meters will give a different result with a different drop of blood. As long as there is not a big difference (more than 2mmol/L) there is not usually cause for concern.

Caring for strips

It is important to care for your strips so that you get an accurate reading. To do this, refer to the manufacturer's instructions. It will include recommendations like:

- Storing them in a dry place
- Replacing the cap immediately after use
- Checking the expiry date is valid.

Bladder & kidneys

Kidney and bladder damage is a complication of diabetes. People with diabetes are at risk of bladder and kidney infections, kidney failure and dialysis. Maintaining good blood glucose control and keeping your blood pressure at a healthy level will reduce this risk. Annual kidney health checks are recommended

Kidney Disease

Kidney disease occurs when the nephrons inside your kidneys, which act as blood filters, are damaged. This leads to the build up of waste and fluids inside the body. If kidney disease is not diagnosed, it can lead to serious complications including kidney failure, which requires dialysis or a kidney transplant to keep you alive.

Kidney disease and diabetes

Each kidney contains up to one million nephrons, the filtering units of the kidneys. Inside a nephron is a tiny set of looping blood vessels called the glomerulus. Diabetes can damage the kidney filters, leading to diabetic kidney disease, or diabetic nephropathy. If kidney disease is found early, medication, dietary and lifestyle changes can increase the life of your kidneys and keep you feeling your best for as long as possible.

Symptoms

In some cases diabetic kidney disease causes the kidney filters to become blocked and stop working, which results in kidney failure. Symptoms of kidney failure may be general and can include:

- changes in the amount and number of times urine is passed
- blood in the urine
- tiredness
- loss of appetite
- difficulty sleeping
- headaches
- lack of concentration
- shortness of breath
- nausea and vomiting

Controlling blood sugar levels can slow down the development of diabetic kidney disease.

Kidney health check

It is very important that diabetic kidney disease is detected early as treatment can help to increase the life of the kidneys. Your health care team can give you practical advice about the best way to keep your kidneys healthy.

If you have diabetes your doctor should undertake a yearly kidney health check, which includes:

- urine test to detect albuminuria
- blood test to estimate the GFR (eGFR)
- blood pressure test

What is albuminuria?

Albumin is a type of protein. The urine test is assessing the rate at which the kidneys are leaking a albumin into the urine. Albuminuria can lead to problems with the body's fluid balance and result in swelling (oedema), often in the legs, feet, face and hands.

The urine is tested with a special test strip in the laboratory. See your doctor immediately if you have any of the above signs of bladder or kidney infection. Any treatment that lowers levels of protein in the urine can help to reduce the rate of progression to kidney failure. ACE inhibitors or ARBs may be used to treat albuminuria. These drugs should be used even if blood pressure is in the desired range.

Being a non-smoker

It is well known that smoking harms the body. Smoking causes a narrowing of the arteries, including the small vessels in the kidney filters. This reduces the kidneys' ability to work properly. If you have diabetes and smoke, the risk of developing albuminuria is much higher. Smoking also increased blood pressure. For reasons that are not well understood, smoking also appears to speed up the progression of diabetic kidney disease to kidney failure.

High blood pressure

Decreasing kidney function is usually linked with a rise in blood pressure. This rise is small at first and may only be detected by taking blood pressure over 24-hours. Even small rises in blood pressure need to be treated, as uncontrolled high blood pressure increases the risk of kidney damage.

If kidney damage is detected, high blood pressure medications called ACE inhibitors (medicines to treat high blood pressure and heart disease) help protect the kidneys from further kidney damage.

Bladder and kidney infection

Bladder and kidney infections are more common in women because of the short length of the urethra, which is the tube taking urine from the bladder to the outside of the body.

The urine and vaginal secretions often contain increased amounts of glucose, particularly if the level of the glucose in the blood has been high. This provides an environment which germs (bacteria and fungi) can grow. It is possible for germs to be forced backwards up this tube during sexual intercourse, so to help prevent infection empty the bladder after sexual intercourse.

If the nerves to the bladder have been damaged by diabetes, the bladder may not empty completely leaving germs that may multiply.

Symptoms and treatment

Prompt treatment of bladder and kidney infections is important. If left untreated may result in chronic kidney damage. In most cases antibiotics taken by mouth effectively treat infections.

If you notice any of the following symptoms of a bladder or kidney infection contact your doctor immediately:

- Passing of small amounts of urine at more frequent intervals, day and night
- A burning discomfort or pain when passing urine
- Backache

This is not an exhaustive list of symptoms and sometimes you may not even have any symptoms at all. If you notice that something isn't right, always check with your doctor.

Diabetes and incontinence type 2 diabetes

If you live with type 2 diabetes, there is potential for your condition to exacerbate any bladder and bowel control problems you may be having.

Being overweight is a condition that puts people at higher risk of both type 2 diabetes and incontinence. Overweight and obesity are major contributors to bladder and bowel control, because the excess strain placed on the pelvic floor muscles weakens them and compromises their ability to support the bladder and bowel, and to shut off the urinary and anal passages.

Fluctuating blood glucose levels or long-term type 2 diabetes can cause damage to nerves, which can lead to problems with bladder and bowel control. This may manifest as a loss in sensation and having little warning about needing to go to the toilet or that your bladder is filling. There may be reduced sensation about whether or not the bladder or bowel is empty, increasing the risk of urinary tract infections (UTIs), kidney damage or constipation.

Diabetes also interferes with the immune system which increases the risk of infection. This combination of immune system decline and poor bladder emptying due to nerve damage, puts people with diabetes at greater risk of UTIs. These can be treated with antibiotics and by practicing good personal hygiene; for example wiping from front to back to avoid contaminating the vagina with bowel bacteria.

The feet (see overleaf).

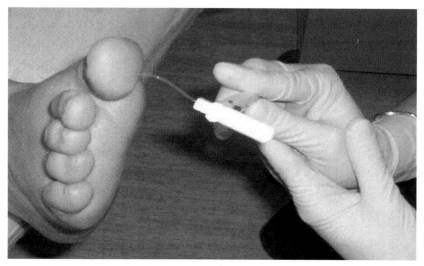

When you have diabetes you need to take care of your feet every day.having diabetes can increase your risk of foot ulcers and amputations and Daily care can prevent serious complications.Check your feet daily for changes or problems and Visit a podiatrist annually for a check up or more frequently if your feet are at high risk

Why?

Your feet are at risk because diabetes can cause damage to the nerves in your feet, blood circulation and infection. Having diabetes can increase your risk of foot ulcers and amputations. This damage is more likely if:

- You have had diabetes for a long time
- Your blood glucose levels have been too high for an extended period

- You smoke – smoking causes a reduced blood flow to your feet, wounds heal slowly
- You are inactive.

Daily checks

It's important to check your feet every day. If you see any of the following- get medical treatment immediatly:

- Ulcer
- Unusual swelling
- Redness
- Blisters
- Ingrown nail
- Bruising or cuts
- Broken skin between toes
- Callus
- Corn
- Foot shape changes
- Cracked skin
- Nail colour changes

Nerve Damage

Poor blood glucose control can cause nerve damage to feet. Symptoms include:

- Numbness
- Coldness of the legs

- A tingling, pins and needles sensation in the feet
- Burning pains in the legs and feet, usually more noticeable in bed at night.

These symptoms can result in a loss of sensation in the feet which increases the risk of accidental damage because you can't feel any pain. An injury to the feet can develop into an ulcer on the bottom of a foot which can penetrate to the bone. This could lead to infection of the bone (osteomyelitis) and a chronic infection in the bones and joints. If an infection isn't treated at the earliest signs, this could result in ulceration (an infected open sore) and eventually amputation (removal of a toe, foot or limb).

Blood Supply

Poor blood glucose control can cause a reduced supply of blood to the feet. This makes people with diabetes more prone to infection following any injury that breaks the skin. Signs of poor blood supply include:

- Sharp leg cramps after walking short distances or up stairs
- Pain in the feet, even at rest (often in the early hours of the morning)
- Feet feeling cold
- Feet looking a reddish-blue colour
- Cuts which are slow to heal.

Checking your feet

There are two types of risk to feet, high risk and low risk. Knowing the risk and taking care of your feet can prevent serious problems like ulcers and amputation. A doctor or podiatrist can carry out an easy and painless check on your feet to determine whether your feet have a low or high risk of developing more serious problems.

Low risk

Low risk feet have normal sensation and good blood flow. However it is important to know that low risk feet can become high risk feet without symptoms, so regular checks are still as important.

High risk

People who have had a foot ulcer or amputation in the past have a high risk of complications. Feet with calluses or deformities like claw toes also have increased risk if poor feeling and/or decreased blood flow are also present.

If your feet are at high risk, you should have them checked by your doctor or a podiatrist every 3 – 6 months. In some cases you may be referred to a specialist or high risk foot clinic. The check-up will include looking at the following:

- Blood flow to the feet (circulation)
- Feeling and reflexes (nerves)

- Unusual foot shapes (including bunions, claw toes and hammer toes)
- Toenails
- Dryness, calluses, corns, cracks or infections.

People with diabetes who have misshapen feet and nerve damage are the more likely to develop:

- Ulcers from too much pressure over some areas of the feet
- More corns and calluses due to too much pressure on one area and can be avoided with some changes.

Seek your podiatrist's help to remove calluses or corns before they become ulcers as these can become infected, risking amputation.

Caring for Your Feet

In addition to regular check-ups with a podiatrist you should also:

- Seek more information about how to care for your feet from a podiatrist
- Have your feet checked at least once a year by your doctor or other health professional
- Know your feet well - wash, dry and check your feet every day. Check for redness, swelling, cuts, pus discharge, splinters or blisters, being especially careful to look between toes, around heels and nail edges and at

the soles of the feet. If you have difficulty with your vision get someone to check for you

- Cut your toenails straight across - not into the corners - and gently file any sharp edges. If you can't properly see or reach your feet to cut your toenails, ask someone to do it for you
- Moisturise your feet daily to avoid dry skin
- Never use over-the-counter corn cures
- Cover your feet with a clean sock or stocking without rough seams
- Don't wear tight socks or stockings
- Protect your feet in a shoe which fits well - the right length (a thumb width longer than your longest toe), width and depth - and has been checked for stones, pins, buttons or anything else which could cause damage
- Keep your feet away from direct heat such as heaters, hot water bottles and electric blankets
- Get medical advice early if you notice any change or problem

Injuries

If you find an injury including a cut, blister, sore, red area or open crack, immediately:

- Wash and dry the area
- Apply good antiseptic e.g. Betadine
- Cover with a sterile dressing, available from pharmacies.

If any injury does not improve within 24 hours, make an urgent appointment to see your doctor to avoid serious complications.

Seek urgent medical advice for even the mildest foot infection, including any sore, open wound or crack which is oozing, contains pus or any type of discharge or which does not heal within a week.

Podiatry

Podiatry is a field of healthcare devoted to the study and treatment of disorders of the foot, ankle, and the knee, leg and hip, collectively known as the lower extremity.

Some health services offer subsidised podiatry services. Phone your local hospital, find out more.

Heart Disease

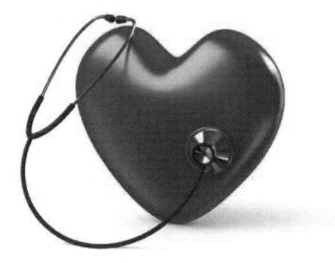

Diabetes puts you at risk of heart disease (even if you have 'normal' looking cholesterol and no symptoms). This is because diabetes can change the chemical makeup of some of the substances found in the blood and this can cause blood vessels to narrow or to clog up completely.

Heart attacks and strokes are up to four times more likely in people with diabetes. For this reason, often people with diabetes are on blood pressure lowering medications, often in combination. Maintaining fitness with regular physical activity combined with some weight loss can help reduce high blood pressure.

Why is there an increased rate of heart disease?

Diabetes can change the chemical makeup of some of the substances found in the blood and this can cause blood vessels to narrow or to clog up completely.

Maintaining fitness with regular physical activity combined with some weight loss can help reduce high blood pressure. Blood pressure lowering medications are often required for people who have diabetes.

Symptoms

Often people do not know they have heart disease until they develop symptoms like chest pain, shortness of breath, dizziness or excessive fatigue when walking or exercising. It is important to note that symptoms may be mild to severe and sometimes there may be none at all. Examples of some other warning symptoms may be arm or jaw discomfort, indigestion, weakness, nausea.

Reducing the risk

One of the most important things to do to reduce the risk of heart disease is to meet with your doctor and/or Credentialled Diabetes Educator to discuss your individual risk factors and how to reduce them. In general terms you can reduce the risk by:

- Being physically active
- Losing weight if you are overweight
- Not smoking
- Managing blood fats
- Managing high blood pressure
- Taking medication as prescribed.

Be physically active

Regular physical activity combined with a healthy diet and achieving/maintaining a healthy weight can help to reduce the risk of a heart attack and stroke. Any type of physical activity– whether sports, household work, gardening or work-related physical activity – will help.

Aim to do at least 30 minutes of moderate intensity physical activity on most, if not all, days of the week. Moderate intensity is when your breathing increases noticeably – a 'little bit of puff'. Check with your doctor before beginning a physical activity program.

Lose weight

Being overweight, especially around waist is a major risk factor for heart disease. Even a 10% weight loss (e.g. a loss of 10 kgs in a 100 kg person) reduces the risk of heart disease.

Don't smoke

Smoking is a very important risk factor for heart disease compared with non-smokers. Stopping smoking at any age can significantly improve health, including reduced risk of heart diseases.

Take medications as prescribed

As cardiovascular disease is the leading cause of death in people with diabetes, statins (medicines that reduce cholesterol) are usually required to manage cholesterol levels to reduce risk. The most recent research indicates that statins should be considered for all adults with diabetes, even those without any signs of heart disease. Medication, referred to as 'blood pressure lowering agents' can also help lower high blood pressure. You may require more than one agent.

Ask your doctor about aspirin to help reduce the risk of heart attack. Aspirin in low doses is sometimes recommended for people at risk of heart attacks as it makes the blood thinner and less likely to clog blood vessels.

Always take your medication as prescribed by your doctor. If you have any concerns then discuss them with doctor, do not alter your medication yourself.

Sexual health

A healthy sexual relationship is one of life's expectations and pleasures. When things go wrong, whether or not we have diabetes, many of us find it hard to accept that there might be a problem. It's important to know there is support available.

While most people with diabetes, both male and female, are able to lead completely normal sex lives, diabetes may contribute to sexual problems for some people. The most common problem is erectile dysfunction in men (also known as impotence) which results in the inability to get or keep an erection long enough for intercourse. Ejaculation may or may not be affected. Fertility remains normal. Both men and women with diabetes may also lose their sexual desire when their blood glucose levels are high.

Erectile dysfunction

Most men have an occasional problem with erectile dysfunction at some time in their life. This can be caused by many factors like being tired, stressed, and depressed or drinking too much alcohol. Some medications may also cause erectile dysfunction, such medications for high blood pressure, depression or stomach ulcers. It's important to always tell your doctor about any medications you may be taking for other conditions.

Reduced blood flow and nerve damage to the penis are generally the underlying reasons for erectile dysfunction for men with diabetes. Often men with diabetes who have the condition also have other complications related to nerve damage or blood circulation problems, such as high blood pressure, high cholesterol or heart disease. Erectile dysfunction can be treated in a number of ways including:

- Tablets (e.g. Viagra, Cialis and Levitra)
- Prostaglandin injection into the side of the penis (e.g. Caverject)
- Devices such as the vacuum pump
- Surgery such as penile implants.

While tablets are easy to take, they may not work for everyone. So discuss all the options with your doctor to decide what's best for you.

Sexual & reproductive health in women

In general, much less is known about sexual problems in women and this includes women with diabetes. The main sexual problems that women deal with are vaginal dryness, a decrease in sexual desire, pain during sex and trouble having an orgasm. Whether diabetes affects these problems is unclear although women who find it hard to come to terms with having diabetes are more likely to report sexual problems.

Women with poorly controlled diabetes are more likely to have frequent bouts of thrush (yeast infection). In most cases, keeping blood glucose levels under control will help.

During periods or menopause, blood glucose levels may change. Women affected by this will need to adjust their treatment. Your doctor will help during these times.

Dealing with sexual problems

Sexual problems are the same as any other medical problem. You need to talk to your doctor about the strategies that will best suit you and your lifestyle.

Accept that there is a problem. Thinking it might go away will only delay treatment. The sooner you seek help the sooner the problem can be treated. If you have a partner, talk through the problems you are both experiencing. Sexual problems have the potential to cause a strain in the relationship. If you feel this is happening, you may like to contact

Diabetes-depression and mental health

Depression is a very real condition and is becoming increasingly common in the general population; approximately one in four people will experience depression some time in their adult life. For people who live with diabetes, this figure is even higher. Up to 50% of people with diabetes are thought to also have a mental illness such as depression or anxiety.

People with depression and diabetes may find it hard to maintain daily diabetes care

What is Depression?

Depression is not just low mood but a serious illness. People with depression find it hard to do normal activities and function from day to day. Depression has serious effects on physical as well as mental health.

Link between diabetes and depression

Research shows that having diabetes more than doubles the risk of developing depression. Living with a chronic condition like diabetes, coping with biological and hormonal factors plus needing to manage the condition on a daily basis may increase the risk of depression.

Depression can increase the likelihood of developing diabetes complications. People with depression may find it harder to deal with everyday tasks. Over time, managing diabetes (regular blood glucose testing, taking medication, following a healthy eating plan and regular physical activity) can take its toll. This may increase a person's risk of depression, which may in turn lead to their usual diabetes care being neglected.

Treatment

Depression is just like any other illness, it can be treated. Treatment can lift the depression and improve diabetes control.

Looking after your diabetes will help decrease the risk of getting depression. If you already have depression, good diabetes management will help lessen the negative impacts it can have. Depression is no different to any of the other complication of diabetes. It is a genuine illness for which you need to seek help and support from health professionals.

The treatment for depression and diabetes involves a coordinated approach that monitors both diabetes control and the symptoms of depression. It is about finding the treatment that works best for each person. For example, people with diabetes and mild depression may find that regular physical activity improves depressed moods and also helps control blood glucose levels.

The most effective treatments combine psychological and medical care. Talk to your doctor about how you are feeling and discuss whether a referral for psychological support is appropriate. Support is vital and can come from a number of sources such as friends, family and community groups Your doctor or health professional will take into account several factors when suggesting the most suitable treatment for you. Regular contact with, and ongoing assessment by your doctor to check that your treatments are working effectively is an important part of becoming and, staying well.

Helping yourself

If you suspect you might have depression, take control of your health by:

- Going to a doctor or other health professional
- Getting involved in social activities
- Engaging in regular moderate physical activity
- Learning about depression and diabetes
- Eating healthily and including a wide variety of foods
- Achieving and maintaining healthy weight
- Limiting your alcohol intake
- Getting help, support and encouragement from family and friends

- Asking your doctor to check your blood pressure, cholesterol and blood glucose levels.

Diabetes UK contains help and advice when dealing with depression and has a list of useful contacts to help you find advice and support if dealing with depression. their website is www.diabetes.org.uk

Diabetes UK also covers a wide range of areas dealing with all aspects of healthcare. They can be contacted on 0345 123 2399, which is a helpline offering help and support on all aspects of diabetes.

Now read the Main Points from chapter 3 overleaf.

****

Main Points from Chapter 3

- The point or aim of all treatment for diabetes is to keep the level of glucose in the bloodstream as close as possible to normal.

- Self-blood glucose monitoring allows you to check your blood glucose levels as often as you need to or as recommended by your doctor.

- Kidney and bladder damage is a complication of diabetes. People with diabetes are at risk of bladder and kidney infections, kidney failure and dialysis. Maintaining good blood glucose control and keeping your blood pressure at a healthy level will reduce this risk. Annual kidney health checks are recommended

- When you have diabetes you need to take care of your feet every day.Having diabetes can increase your risk of foot ulcers and amputations and Daily care can prevent serious complications.Check your feet daily for changes or problems and Visit a podiatrist annually for a check up or more frequently if your feet are at high risk

- Diabetes puts you at risk of heart disease (even if you have 'normal' looking cholesterol and no symptoms). This is because diabetes can change the chemical makeup of some of the substances found in the blood and this can cause blood vessels to narrow or to clog up completely.

- A healthy sexual relationship is one of life's expectations and pleasures. When things go wrong, whether or not we have diabetes, many of us find it hard to accept that there might be a problem. It's important to know there is support available.

- Up to 50% of people with diabetes are thought to also have a mental illness such as depression or anxiety.

****

Chapter 4

The Importance of Diet and Exercise

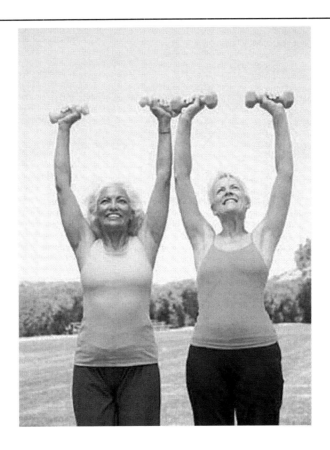

Diabetes and Exercise

People with diabetes are encouraged to exercise regularly for better blood sugar control and to reduce the risk of cardiovascular diseases. The reason for this is that muscles which are working use more glucose than those that are resting.

Muscle movement leads to greater sugar uptake by muscle cells and lower blood sugar levels.

Additional benefits of exercise include a healthier heart, better weight control and stress management.

The Importance of exercise

As well as strengthening the cardiovascular system and the body's muscles, many people exercise to keep fit, lose or maintain a healthy weight, sharpen their athletic skills, or purely for enjoyment. Regular, frequent physical exercise is recommended for people of all age groups as it boosts the immune system and helps to protect against conditions such as:

- Heart disease
- Stroke
- Type 2 diabetes
- Cancer and other major illnesses

In fact, it is known to cut your risk of major chronic illnesses/diseases by up to 50% and reduce your risk of early death by up to 30%. There are other health benefits of exercising on a regular basis which include:

- Improvements in mental health
- It boosts self-esteem/confidence
- It enhances sleep quality and energy levels
- It cuts risk of stress and depression
- It protects against dementia and alzheimer's disease

Defining exercise

In the UK, regular exercise is defined by the NHS as completing 150 minutes of moderate intensity aerobic activity a week. Aerobic activity at moderate intensity means exercising at a level that raises your heart rate and makes you sweat. This includes a multitude of sports. For example;

- Walking at a fast pace
- Jogging lightly
- Bike riding
- Rowing
- Playing tennis or badminton
- Water aerobics

The less time you spend sitting down, the better it will be for your health. Sedentary behaviour, such as sitting or lying down for long periods, increases your risk of weight gain and obesity, which in turn, may also up your risk of chronic diseases such as heart disease.

Taking precautions

There are precautions which people with diabetes must take when exercising. Exercise precautions are designed to help people with diabetes avoid problems which can result from unwise exercise choices.

Hypoglycemia can occur if a person who is taking blood sugar lowering medication has:

- Eaten too little carbohydrate (fruit, milk, starch) relative to the exercise.
- Taken too much medication relative to the exercise
- Combined effect of food and medication imbalances relative to the exercise

Those who do not take diabetes medication do not need to take these precautions. Drink plenty of water before, during and after exercise to stay well hydrated.

Precautions for people on insulin or oral medication

Precautions to take if you take insulin or oral diabetes medication:

- If your blood sugar level is less than 5.5 mmols/l (100 mg/dl) prior to exercise, take a carbohydrate snack prior to beginning the exercise.
- If your blood sugar level is higher than 5.5 mmols/l (100 mg/dl) before exercise, it may not be necessary to take a carbohydrate snack before a light exercise session, but you may need extra carbohydrates during or following the exercise. Check your blood to see if your blood sugar dips below 4 mmols/l (70 mg/dl) following exercise.
- If you experience hypoglycemia, follow the Carbohydrate Treatment guidelines. Follow up with your doctor. You may be advised to lower your medication on days you exercise if your blood sugar levels are well-controlled and usually within target range.

- For long duration and/or high intensity exercise sessions, plan extra carbohydrate snacks during the activity. Additional carbohydrates is suggested each 30 to 60 minutes of exercise (e.g. soccer game, hiking, biking, skating, etc).
- Always carry a fast-acting carbohydrate food such as glucose tablets when exercising in the event blood sugar drops too low and hypoglycemia symptoms develop during exercise.
- Wear a form of ID, which identifies you as having diabetes, particularly if you are exercising alone so that others may help you appropriately in the event something unexpected happens.

Diabetes and diet

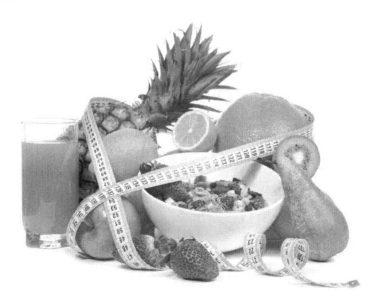

It is a fact that eating well is important, whether or not a person has diabetes. The foods you choose to eat in your daily diet make a difference not only to managing diabetes, but also to how well you feel and how much energy you have every day. How much you need to eat and drink is based on your age, gender, how active you are and the goals you are looking to achieve.

Portion sizes have grown in recent years, as the plates and bowls we use have got bigger. Use smaller crockery to cut back on your portion sizes, while making the food on your plate look bigger. No single food contains all the essential nutrients you need in the right proportion. That's why you need to consume foods from each of the main food groups to eat well.

Fruit and vegetables

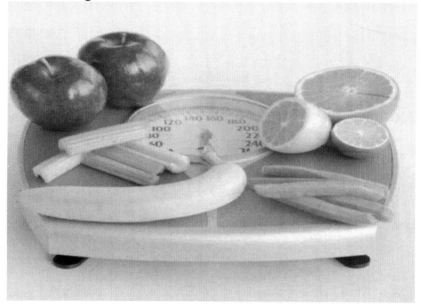

Naturally low in fat and calories and packed full of vitamins, minerals and fibre, fruit and vegetables add flavour and variety to every meal. They may also help protect against stroke, heart disease, high blood pressure and some cancers.

Everyone should eat at least five portions a day. Fresh, frozen, dried and canned fruit in juice and canned vegetables in water all count. Go for a rainbow of colours to get as wide a range of vitamins and minerals as possible. Try:

- adding an apple, banana, pear, or orange to your child's lunchbox
- sliced melon or grapefruit topped with low-fat yogurt, or a handful of berries, or fresh dates, apricots or prunes for breakfast
- carrots, peas and green beans mixed up in a pasta bake
- adding an extra handful of vegetables to your dishes when cooking – peas to rice, spinach to lamb or onions to chicken.

Starchy foods (see overleaf)

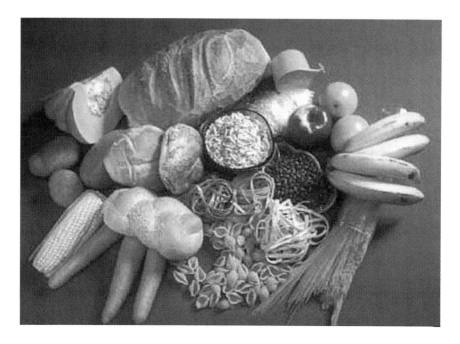

Potatoes, rice, pasta, bread, chapattis, naan and plantain all contain carbohydrate, which is broken down into glucose and used by your cells as fuel.

Better options of starchy foods – such as wholegrain bread, wholewheat pasta and basmati, brown or wild rice – contain more fibre, which helps to keep your digestive system working well. They are generally more slowly absorbed (that is, they have a lower glycaemic index, or GI), keeping you feeling fuller for longer.

Try to include some starchy foods every day.

Try:

- two slices of multigrain toast with a scraping of spread and Marmite or peanut butter

- rice, pasta or noodles in risottos, salads or stir-fries
- potatoes any way you like – but don't fry them – with the skin left on for valuable fibre. Choose low-fat toppings, such as cottage cheese or beans
- baked sweet potato, with the skin left on for added fibre
- boiled cassava, flavoured with chilli and lemon
- chapatti made with brown or wholemeal atta.

Meat, fish, eggs, pulses, beans and nuts

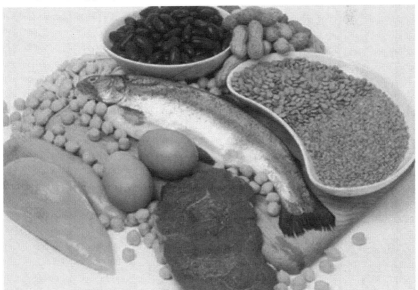

These foods are high in protein, which helps with building and replacing muscles. They contain minerals, such as iron, which are vital for producing red blood cells. Oily fish, such as mackerel, salmon and sardines, also provide omega-3, which can help protect the heart. Beans, pulses, soya and tofu are also good sources of protein.

Aim to have some food from this group every day, with at least 1–2 portions of oily fish a week.

Try:

- serving meat, poultry or a vegetarian alternative grilled, roasted or stir-fried
- a small handful of raw nuts and seeds as a snack or chopped with a green salad
- using beans and pulses in a casserole to replace some – or all – of the meat
- grilled fish with masala, fish pie, or make your own fish cakes
- eggs scrambled, poached, dry fried or boiled – the choice is yours!

Dairy foods (overleaf)

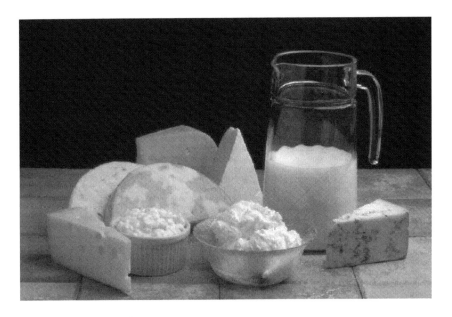

Milk, cheese and yogurt contain calcium, which is vital for growing children as it keeps their bones and teeth strong. They're good sources of protein, too.

Some dairy foods are high in fat, particularly saturated fat, so choose lower-fat alternatives (check for added sugar, though). Semi-skimmed milk actually contains more calcium than whole milk, but children under 2 should have whole milk because they may not get the calories or essential vitamins they need from lower-fat milks. Don't give children skimmed milk until they're at least 5. Aim to have some dairy every day, but don't overdo it.

Try:

- milk straight in a glass, flavoured with a little cinnamon, or added to breakfast porridge

- yogurt with fruit or on curry
- cottage cheese scooped on carrot sticks
- a bowl of breakfast cereal in the morning, with skimmed or semi-skimmed milk
- a cheese sandwich at lunchtime, packed with salad
- a refreshing lassi or some plain yogurt with your evening meal.

Foods high in fat and sugar

You can enjoy food from this group as an occasional treat in a balanced diet, but remember that sugary foods and drinks will add extra calories – and sugary drinks will raise blood glucose – so opt for diet/light or low-calorie alternatives. Or choose water – it's calorie free!

Fat is high in calories, so try to reduce the amount of oil or butter you use in cooking. Remember to use unsaturated oils, such as sunflower, rapeseed or olive oil, as these types are better for your heart.

Salt

Too much salt can make you more at risk of high blood pressure and stroke. Processed foods can be very high in salt. Try cooking more meals from scratch at home, where you can control the amount of salt you use – when there are so many delicious spices in your kitchen, you really can enjoy your favourite recipes with less salt.

Adults should have no more than 1 tsp (6g) of salt a day, while children have even lower targets.

Try:
- banishing the salt cellar from the table, but keeping the black pepper.
- seasoning food with herbs and spices, instead of salt. Try ginger, lime and coriander in stir-fries, or use spicy harissa paste to flavour soups, pasta dishes and couscous.
- making fresh chutney using coriander leaves (dhaniya), fresh mint, chopped green chillies and lime juice.
- measuring added salt in cooking with a teaspoon and use less as time goes on. Do it gradually, and the family will hardly notice!
- flavouring salads with lemon juice, chilli powder and pepper.
- making your own tandoori marinade in seconds using red chilli powder, ground garam masala, paprika powder, low-fat plain yogurt, garlic, ginger, and tomato purée.
- adding finely chopped coriander leaves to lassi, and sprinkle on ground jeera and ground coriander seeds.

Type 1 diabetes and coeliac disease

This is an autoimmune disease, which is more common in people with Type 1 diabetes, where the body reacts to gluten (a protein found in wheat, barley and rye), which damages the gut lining and makes it difficult to absorb food.

Everyone with Type 1 diabetes should be assessed for coeliac disease. If you are showing symptoms, you should be given a blood test. If the test is positive, diagnosis is confirmed by a gut biopsy. Don't start a gluten-free diet until you have a definite diagnosis, as this may give an inaccurate result. The only treatment is to cut out gluten from your diet permanently. A specialist dietitian can help you with both diabetes and coeliac disease.

Natural remedies and diabetes

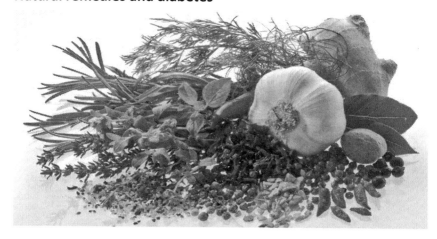

Many common herbs and spices are claimed to have blood sugar lowering properties that make them useful for people with or at high risk of type 2 diabetes. A number of clinical studies have been carried out in recent years that show potential links between herbal therapies and improved blood glucose control, which has led to an increase in people with diabetes using these more 'natural' ingredients to help manage their condition.

Plant-based therapies that have been shown in some studies to have anti-diabetic properties include:

- Aloe vera
- Bilberry extract
- Bitter melon
- Cinnamon
- Fenugreek
- Ginger
- Okra

While such therapies are commonly used in ayurvedic and oriental medicine for treating serious conditions such as diabetes, many health experts in the west remain sceptical about their reported medical benefits.

If you decide to follow a particular dietary path then it is important that you first discuss this with your doctor.

Aloe Vera and Diabetes

Aloe vera is a product of the prickly and succulent aloe vera plant, which has been used in herbal medicine for thousands of years due to its healing, rejuvenating and soothing properties. Native to the Caribbean, South Africa and Latin America, the plant's leaves contain a clear gel that is widely used in Creams, lotions, shampoos and ointments

Preliminary research suggests that intake of aloe vera juice can help improve blood glucose levels and may therefore be useful in treating people with diabetes. Aloe has also been linked with:

- Decreased blood lipids (fats) in patients with abnormally high levels of these molecules in the blood (e.g. some people with type 2 diabetes) and/or acute hepatitis (liver disease)

- Decreased swelling and faster healing of wound injuries. Leg wounds and ulcers are common complications of diabetes, and they typically take longer time to heal than in healthy non-diabetic individuals. [67]

These positive effects are thought to be due to the presence of compounds such as lectins, mannans and anthraquinones.

Bilberry extract

Bilberries (scientific name: vaccinium myrtillus) are a dark blue fruit, similar in appearance to blueberries but are smaller, softer and darker. Studies indicate that a compound in bilberries, anthocyanosides, appear to promote blood vessel strength which could have protective properties against forms of retinal damage in people with diabetes.

Bilberry extract and retinopathy

Retinopathy and maculopathy are both conditions of the retina in the eye that are more likely to develop in people with diabetes. Research has shown that people with retinopathy that took bilberry extract during the study showed signs of strengthening of blood vessels in the retina and reduced haemorrhaging. The research that has been carried out to date has been small scale and so whilst bilberry extract shows promise, researchers are yet to find out how much bilberry extract may be of help in limiting the development of retinopathy.

Bilberries and lower blood glucose levels

Bilberry extract is not recognised as a treatment for diabetes but people with diabetes may notice that it helps in lowering blood glucose levels. If you are on blood glucose lowering medication that can bring on hypoglycemia, you may need to monitor your blood glucose levels and take precautions to ensure blood sugar levels don't go too low.

Bitter Melon and Diabetes

Bitter melon, also known as bitter gourd or karela (in India), is a unique vegetable-fruit that can be used as food or medicine. It is the edible part of the plant Momordica Charantia, which is a vine of the Cucurbitaceae family and is considered the most bitter among all fruits and vegetables.

The bitter melon itself grows off the vine as a green, oblong-shaped fruit with a distinct warty exterior - though its size, texture and bitterness vary between the different regions in which it grows - and is rich in vital vitamins and minerals.

In addition to being a food ingredient, bitter melon has also long been used as a herbal remedy for a range of ailments, including type 2 diabetes. The fruit contains at least three active substances with anti-diabetic properties, including charantin, which has been confirmed to have a blood glucose-lowering effect, vicine and an insulin-like compound known as polypeptide-p.

These substances either work individually or together to help reduce blood sugar levels. It is also known that bitter melon contains a lectin that reduces blood glucose concentrations by acting on peripheral tissues and suppressing appetite - similar to the effects of insulin in the brain. This lectin is thought to be a major factor behind the hypoglycemic effect that develops after eating bitter melon.

Cinnamon and Diabetes

Cinnamon is a sweet but pungent spice that is derived from the inner bark of the branches of wild cinnamon trees, which grow in tropical areas across Southeast Asia, South America and the Caribbean. The use of cinnamon dates back thousands of years and was highly prized among many ancient civilisations.

Cinnamon, often used in cooking and baking, is increasingly being linked to improvements in the treatment of conditions such as diabetes mellitus. Research has suggested that cinnamon can help to improve blood glucose levels and increase insulin sensitivity.

Results from a clinical study published in the *Diabetes Care* journal in 2003 suggest that cassia cinnamon (cinnamon bark) improves blood glucose and cholesterol levels in people with type 2 diabetes, and may reduce risk factors associated with diabetes and cardiovascular disease.

A daily intake of just 1, 3, or 6 grams was shown to reduce serum glucose, triglyceride, LDL or bad cholesterol and total cholesterol after 40 days among 60 middle-aged diabetics.

Health benefits of cinnamon

In addition to regulating blood glucose and lowering cholesterol, cinnamon has been shown to:

- Have an anti-clotting effect on the blood
- Relieve pain in arthritis sufferers
- Boost the body's immune system
- Stop medication-resistant yeast infections
- Help in relieving indigestion
- Reduce the proliferation of leukaemia and lymphoma cancer cells
- Preserve food by inhibiting bacterial growth and food spoilage
- Be a great source of vital nutrients, including calcium, fibre, manganese and iron

The majority of these health benefits are associated with use of true cinnamon (also known as Ceylon cinnamon) and not cassia bark cinnamon, which is the species involved in most diabetes research.

Fenugreek and Diabetes

Fenugreek is an aromatic plant that has many uses, both culinary fenugreek is a key ingredient of curries and other Indian recipes and medicinal. The plant, which is widely grown in South Asia, North Africa and parts of the Mediterranean, has small round leaves and also produces long pods that contain distinctive bitter-tasting seeds.

The leaves are either sold as a vegetable (fresh leaves, sprouts, and microgreens) commonly known as methi, or as an herb (dried leaves), while the seeds are used both whole and in powdered form as a spice.

As well as being a popular cooking ingredient, fenugreek has a number of health benefits and is used in both Ayurvedic and traditional Chinese medicine.

Fenugreek seeds (trigonella foenum graecum) are high in soluble fibre, which helps lower blood sugar by slowing down digestion and absorption of carbohydrates. This suggests they may be effective in treating people with diabetes. Studies have been carried out to investigate the potential anti-diabetic benefits of fenugreek. Of these, several clinical trials showed that fenugreek seeds can improve most metabolic symptoms associated with both type 1 and type 2 diabetes in humans by lowering blood glucose levels and improving glucose tolerance.

Ginger and Diabetes

Ginger is the thick knotted underground stem (rhizome) of the plant Zingiber officinale that has been used for centuries in Asian cuisine and medicine. Native to Africa, India, China, Australia and Jamaica, it is commonly used as a spice or flavouring agent in cooking, as an alternative 'herbal' treatment for various ailments such as nausea and indigestion, and for fragrance in soaps and cosmetics.

Ginger rhizome can be used fresh, dried and powdered, or as a juice or oil. It has a pungent and sharp aroma and adds a strong spicy flavour to food and drink.

Insulin secretion

In the December 2009 issue of the European Journal of Pharmacology, researchers reported that two different ginger extracts, spissum and an oily extract, interact with serotonin receptors to reveres their effect on insulin secretion.

Treatment with the extracts led to a 35 per cent drop in blood glucose levels and a 10 per cent increase in plasma insulin levels.

Cataract protection

A study published in the August 2010 edition of Molecular Vision revealed that a small daily dose of ginger helped delay the onset and progression of cataracts - one of the sight-related complications of long-term diabetes - in diabetic rats.

It's also worth noting that ginger has a very low glycemic index (GI). Low GI foods break down slowly to form glucose and therefore do not trigger a spike in blood sugar levels as high GI foods do.

Ginger has been used as an herbal therapy in Chinese, Indian, and Arabic medicine for centuries to aid digestion, combat the common cold and relieve pain.

Its powerful anti-inflammatory substances, gingerols, make it an effective pain reliever and it is commonly used to reduce pain and swelling in patients with arthritis and those suffering from other inflammation and muscle complaints.

In fact, ginger is said to be just as effective as nonsteroidal anti-inflammatory drugs, but without the gastro-intestinal side effects. Other medical uses of ginger include treatment of:

- Bronchitis
- Heartburn
- Menstrual pain
- Nausea and vomiting
- Upset stomach
- Diarrhoea
- Upper respiratory tract infections (URTI)

Okra

Commonly referred to as ladyfingers, or by its biological names Abelmoschus esculentus and Hibiscus esculentus, okra is known to have a positive effect on blood sugar control, among many other health benefits.

Okra is a tall-growing vegetable that traces its origin from ancient Ethiopia (Abyssinia) through to Eastern Mediterranean,

India, the Americas and the Caribbean. Parts of the plant (immature okra pods) are widely used vegetables in tropical countries and are typically used for making soups, stews or as a fried/boiled vegetable.

These tender pods are very low in calories, providing just 30 calories per 100 g, and contain no saturated fats or cholesterol. They are also rich in nutrients, completely non-toxic, and have no adverse side effects.

Evidence of okra having anti-diabetic properties has increased in recent years, with multiple Vitro (laboratory) and Vivo (animal) studies confirming okra as a potent blood glucose-lowering (or anti-diabetic) food.

Because okra is a rich source of dietary fibre, important vitamins and minerals, and powerful antioxidants, the vegetable is known to be beneficial for health in a number of ways. These include:

- Preventing and improving constipation
- Lowering cholesterol
- Reducing the risk of some forms of cancer, especially colorectal cancer
- Improving energy levels and improving symptoms of depression
- Helping to treat sore throat, irritable bowel, ulcers and lung inflammation

Now read the Main Points from Chapter 4

****

Main Points from Chapter 4

- People with diabetes are encouraged to exercise regularly for better blood sugar control and to reduce the risk of cardiovascular diseases. The reason for this is that muscles which are working use more glucose than those that are resting. Muscle movement leads to greater sugar uptake by muscle cells and lower blood sugar levels. Additional benefits of exercise include a healthier heart, better weight control

- It is a fact that eating well is important, whether or not a person has diabetes. The foods you choose to eat in your daily diet make a difference not only to managing diabetes, but also to how well you feel and how much energy you have every day. How much you need to eat and drink is based on your age, gender, how active you are and the goals you are looking to achieve.

****

Chapter 5

Medication and Diabetes

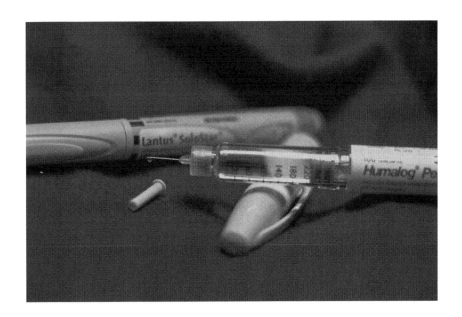

Insulin

For Diabetes 1, or for those with diabetes 2 who are not responding to oral medication, insulin is the only effective medication. There is only one effective way of getting it into the bloodstream, that is by injection. If it is swallowed it is only part digested and therefore its job cannot be done properly.

Insulin is usually injected under the skin as opposed to through a vein or into a muscle. It would be injected into a vein or muscle only in special circumstances, such as if you were ill or having an operation.

Types of insulin

Insulin is divided into short, medium or longer-term varieties, with the difference being how long they take to take effect. Short-acting insulin is always clear and without colour, whereas the other two can be cloudy because they may contain additives to slow down the absorption of insulin from under the skin. There are ready mixed kinds on the market that will save you the trouble of mixing them yourself.

Insulin is generally produced from animal sources-pig or beef-or from genetically engineered human hormone. New technology is enabling scientists to produce insulins from genetic technology. These insulins, called analogues, are absorbed either more quickly or more slowly and smoothly. Quick acting analogues can be injected immediately before or during a meal (or even after) and are therefore more convenient for those people with variable mealtimes.

There are three long-acting insulins available in the UK at the moment, glargine, detemir and degludec. These insulins can be given once or twice daily at any time but should be taken at the same time each day.

The aim of insulin therapy

The main objective of insulin therapy is to imitate the body's natural supply as closely as possible. In a person who doesn't have diabetes, insulin is released by the pancreas in response to food. As the blood glucose levels fall between meals, so the insulin levels drop back towards zero. It never quite reaches zero and at all times there is detectable insulin in the bloodstream. What you are trying to do when you give yourself insulin injections is to reproduce the normal pattern of insulin production from the pancreas.

There are several ways to achieve this using different types of insulin and numbers of injections each day. One example is people sticking to a routine such as three short-acting injections per day before a meal and then one night-time injection of a longer acting insulin to control blood glucose whilst they are sleeping. This is called a 'basal-bolus' regime and is currently recommended for all type 1 diabetes.

Another system, quite popular, involves two injections per day of a mixture of short and medium acting insulins. The short-acting component covers the meal that you are about to have (say breakfast or evening meal) whilst the medium acting component covers you at lunchtime or overnight.

Your diabetes nurse will help you with the process of injections, where and how you inject yourself. Most people use disposable syringes, as they minimise the risk of infection.

There are also insulin injection pens, which are quite popular, largely due to their portability. They have now mainly replaced syringes and the pens and needles are available on prescription.

Insulin pumps

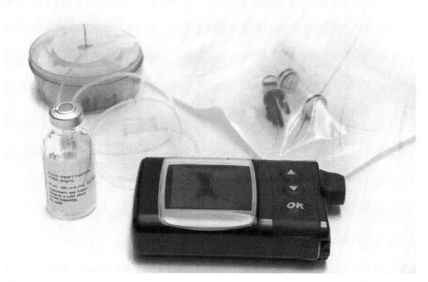

Although the main way of injecting insulin is via a needle, some people have found that giving insulin by a pump which provides a constant infusion, like drip feeding, under the skin via a thin plastic tube and needle gives smoother blood glucose control. They can be adjusted if the blood glucose levels are too high or too low. However, they require patients to test their blood at least four times a day and therefore it is a more exacting regime. Pumps will be suitable for certain types of people, such as adults with irregular lifestyles but they are expensive (around £3,000) and cost quite a lot to run.

Insulin passports

Insulin passports are a new initiative in the UK, from the NHS and promoted by Diabetes UK, to help people who take insulin to get the right type and dose of insulin. This is very useful in the case of an emergency, such as being taken to hospital or a wrongly made-up prescription. The passport can be kept in a wallet and is feely available from pharmacies or surgeries. It can be used to record:

- Up to date details of the type of insulin, syringes and pens that you use
- Emergency information that tells people what to do if you are found ill or unconscious; and
- Other information to help in an emergency, including contact names and telephone numbers and other medication that you may be taking

How to use your Insulin Passport for greater safety.

- Know the details of the type of insulin you use, and the pen, syringes and other equipment that you use
- Record this information yourself in your Insulin Passport
- Keep it up to date. Whenever your insulin type changes draw a single line through the old information, so that new information can be clearly seen
- There is an option to record other medication that you take
- When you need a new passport see your GP or practice nurse for a new one
- Include information on what you want people to do if you need help with a low blood glucose level (or hypoglycaemic event)

- Keep your credit card sized Insulin Passport somewhere easy to find in an emergency, like your wallet or purse.

Type 2 diabetes

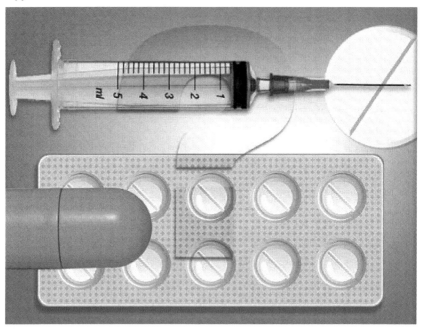

For those with type 2 diabetes, there are seven different kinds of tablets and one injection treatment, as follows:

- o Sulfonylureas
- o Biguanides
- o Acarbose
- o Thiazolidinediones
- o Glinides
- o Gliptines
- o Sodium-glucose 2 (SGLT2) Inhibitors

As usual, they have long and convoluted names, but they all come under one general name of oral hypoglyceamic agents (OHA's). The tablets can be taken alone as part of prescribed medicine or as a combination.

The above medication, either as a single prescription or a combination, together with a healthy lifestyle, diet and exercise, will keep diabetes under control. As is the norm with medication, it can sometimes take a while to arrive at the right combination. Your GP will experiment with this.

We should look below at each of the above medicines and how they work.

Sulphonylureas

Sulphonylureas are a class of oral (tablet) medications that control blood sugar levels in patients with type 2 diabetes by stimulating the production of insulin in the pancreas and increasing the effectiveness of insulin in the body. They are generally taken once or twice a day, with or shortly before a meal, and can be taken on their own or prescribed for use alongside other diabetes drugs such as metformin.

The following drugs are all in the sulphonylureas class (trade name first, generic name in brackets):

- Amaryl (Glimepiride)
- Daonil (Gilbenclamide)
- Diamicron (Gilclazide)
- Diamicron MR (Gilclazide)
- Glibenese (Gilpizide)

- Minodiab (Gilpizide)
- Tolbutamide (Tolbutamide)

Sulphonylureas are insulin secretagogues, which means they work by causing the body to secrete insulin. Sulphonylureas bind to a channel of proteins in the pancreas (ATP-sensitive potassium channel). This triggers a sequence of events within the cells that leads to an increase in the amount of insulin that is produced by pancreatic beta cells.

Sulphonylureas are suitable for people with type 2 diabetes with blood glucose levels that are higher than the recommended levels (an HbA1c above 6.5%) usually once metformin has been prescribed. Sulphonylureas are not appropriate for people with significantly diminished ability to produce insulin, such as those with type 1 diabetes or that have had a pancreatectomy.

The primary benefit of sulphonylureas is their effect on increasing insulin secretion and therefore helping to reduce blood glucose levels. Sulphonylureas are not recommended for people who are overweight or obese, as their mode of action (increase in insulin production and secretion) means that weight gain can be a relatively common side effect. Their effect on insulin levels also means users are at increased risk of hypoglycaemia (low blood sugar), although this risk is reduced with newer sulphonylureas such as glimepiride.

In addition, some users may suffer an allergic reaction during the first six weeks to eight weeks of treatment, resulting in itchy red skin/skin rashes. If this happens, you might need to switch to another anti-diabetes drug.

Biguanides

Biguanide refers to a group of oral type 2 diabetes drugs that work by preventing the production of glucose in the liver, improving the body's sensitivity towards insulin and reducing the amount of sugar absorbed by the intestines.

The only available biguanide medication is metformin, which is commonly used as a first-line treatment for type 2 diabetes (i.e. the first option for type 2 diabetics who are unable to control their blood sugars through diet and exercise alone). Metformin is usually prescribed as a single treatment (monotherapy), but it can also be combined with other medication in a single tablet - for example, metformin + pioglitazone (Competact), metformin + vildagliptin (Eucreas) and metformin + sitagliptin (Janumet). It's also sometimes prescribed in combination with insulin for people with type 1 diabetes.

There are two different versions of the drug;

- Metformin IR (immediate release) - taken up to three times a day
- Metformin SR (slow release) - usually taken once per day

Biguanides work by preventing the liver from converting fats and amino-acids into glucose. They also activate an enzyme (AMPK) which helps cells to respond more effectively to insulin and take in glucose from the blood.

Metformin is generally suitable for most people with type 2 diabetes as a first line of medication if lifestyle changes have no sufficiently lowered blood glucose levels. Metformin can be taken on its own, or in addition to other oral or injectable diabetes medications. It may also be prescribed in combination with insulin for people with type 1 diabetes who have signs of insulin resistance. By reducing the liver's blood glucose raising effect, metformin helps to lower blood glucose levels through the day. Rather than stimulating the release of insulin, metformin increases the body's sensitivity to insulin and therefore has benefits for weight management.

As a monotherapy, metformin users are unlikely to experience hypoglycemia or weight gain. However, the risk of these side effects increases if the drug is taken together with insulin or a sulphonylurea.

Acarbose-Thiazolidinediones (Glitazones)

Thiazolidinediones, also known as glitazones, are a group of oral anti-diabetic drugs designed to treat patients with type 2 diabetes. Classed as oral hypoglycemic drugs along with biguanides, they are taken once or twice daily with or without food and work by targeting insulin resistance - a core physiologic defect in those with type 2 diabetes.

By reducing the body's resistance to insulin, the hormone is allowed to work more effectively at improving blood glucose control. Glitazones also help lower blood pressure and improve lipid metabolism by increasing levels of HDL (or 'good') cholesterol and reducing reducing levels.

Drugs in this class

Pioglitazone (Actos) is the only drug in this group available in the UK, following the European ban on rosiglitazone (Avandia). The tablet improves insulin sensitivity and also helps to protect the insulin-producing cells in the pancreas. It can be used on its own as a monotherapy or as combination treatment with either a sulphonylurea or metformin, or insulin.

TZDs work by targeting the PPAR-gamma receptor, which activates a number of genes in the body and plays an important role in how the body metabolises glucose and how the body stores fat. TZDs can therefore help boost insulin sensitivity and preserve the function of insulin producing cells, but they do raise the risk of weight gain.

A thiazolidinedione treatment may be prescribed as a treatment for people with type 2 diabetes if metformin and either sulphonylureas or prandial glucose regulators are not tolerated or successful in lowering blood glucose levels sufficiently. An alternative treatment such as a DPP-4 inhibitor or incretin mimetic may be prescribed if weight gain could present notable health problems.

The benefits of glitazones include decreased blood glucose levels and preservation of the pancreas's ability to produce sufficient levels of insulin. Glitazones also help lower blood pressure and improve lipid metabolism by increasing levels of HDL (or 'good') cholesterol and reducing levels of triglycerides - a type of fat in the bloodstream and fat tissue.

Glinides

Prandial glucose regulators, also known as glinides, are a family of oral medicines developed for the treatment of people with type 2 diabetes mellitus. They are taken up to three times a day prior to meals – up to 30 minutes before eating - in order to limit subsequent post-meal spikes in blood glucose levels. The way they achieve this is by stimulating the pancreatic beta cells to produce more insulin for the body – similar to sulphonylureas.

Prandial glucose regulators have a relatively rapid-onset, but unlike sulphonylureas only last for a short time. There are currently two products classed as prandial glucose regulators (trade name first, generic name in brackets):

- Prandin (Repaglinide)
- Starlix (Nateglinide)

Prandial glucose regulators cause the pancreas to release more of the blood sugar-regulating hormone insulin. Another class of drug that works this way is the sulphonylureas drug class. Prandial glucose regulators work by binding to a channel of proteins (ATP-sensitive potassium channel) in the insulin-producing cells of the pancreas (beta cells). The end result is that the insulin producing beta cells are able to produce more insulin.

The way prandial glucose regulators work is very similar to the function of sulphonylureas, but the different drug classes target different sites and the result is that prandial glucose regulators are able to act quicker than sulphonylureas.

Prandial glucose regulators are suitable for people with type 2 diabetes with blood glucose levels above the NICE guideline target of 6.5%.

Adverse effects of glinides can include:

- hypoglycemia
- allergic skin reactions
- liver problems
- abdominal pain
- nausea
- diarrhoea
- constipation

Gliptins

Dipeptidyl peptidase-4 (DPP-4) inhibitors are a relatively new class of oral diabetes drugs. Also known as gliptins, they are usually prescribed for people with type 2 diabetes who have not responded well to drugs such as metformin and sulphonylureas. DPP-4 inhibitors may help with weight loss as well as decreasing blood glucose levels, but have been linked with higher rates of pancreatitis.

This drug class includes the following medications (trade name first, generic name in brackets):

- Januvia (Sitagliptin)
- Galvus (Vildagliptin)
- Onglyza (Saxagliptin)
- Tradjenta (Linagliptin) – approved for use in the USA

They work by blocking the action of DPP-4, an enzyme which destroys a group of gastrointestinal hormones called incretins. Incretins help stimulate the production of insulin when it is needed (e.g. after eating) and reduce the production of glucagon by the liver when it is not needed (e.g. during digestion). They also slow down digestion and decrease appetite. So by protecting incretins from damage, DPP-4 inhibitors help regulate blood glucose levels.

DPP-4 inhibitors may be used as a second or third line medication for people with type 2 diabetes after prescribing metformin and sulphonylureas, and as an alternative to thiazolidinedione medication. Gliptins are effective in lowering blood glucose levels and, because they can help reduce appetite, may be beneficial for people needing to lose weight.

Adverse effects of DPP-4 inhibitors include:

- gastrointestinal problems – including nausea, diarrhoea and stomach pain
- flu-like symptoms – headache, runny nose, sore throat
- skin reactions – painful skin followed by a red or purple rash

If you have a reaction which causes difficulty breathing or a severe skin reaction, call for medical help.

DPP-4 inhibitors have been linked with an increased risk of pancreatitis. If you experience a severe pain in your upper abdomen which may be accompanied with nausea and/or vomiting, you should seek for medical help.

SGLT2 Inhibitors (Gliflozins)

Sodium-glucose co-transporter-2 (SGLT2) inhibitors are a relatively new group of oral medications used for treating type 2 diabetes. The drugs work by helping the kidneys to lower blood glucose levels. They are taken once a day with or without food.

The following drugs belong to the SGLT2 inhibitors class (trade name first, generic name in brackets):

- Forxiga (Dapagliflozin)
- Invokana (Canagliflozin)
- Jardiance (Empagliflozin)

As of April 2013, dapagliflozin has been approved by NHS Scotland for prescribing in certain people with type 2 diabetes, while canagliflozin has been approved by the FDA for use in the United States.

SGLT2 inhibitors work by preventing the kidneys from reabsorbing glucose back into the blood.

This allows the kidneys to lower blood glucose levels and the excess glucose in the blood is removed from the body via urine.

SGLT2 inhibitors may be suitable for people with type 2 diabetes that have high blood glucose levels despite being on a medication regimen such as metformin and insulin. SGLT2 inhibitors are not recommended for prescribing to people with kidney disease (nephropathy) as kidney disease prevents the drug from working sufficiently well.

SGLT2 inhibitors help to remove glucose from the blood and therefore help to lower blood glucose levels. By removing glucose from the body, SGLT2 inhibitors can also have benefits for weight loss.

As the drugs cause more glucose to be excreted in the urine, there is a higher chance of getting genital and urinary tract infections. These side effects are more common in women than in men. Patients taking SGLT2 inhibitors with insulin should be aware of the risks of hypoglycemia.

Incretin Mimetics (GLP-1 Agonists)

Incretin mimetics are a relatively new group of injectable drugs for treatment of type 2 diabetes. The drugs, also commonly known as glucagon-like peptide 1 (GLP-1) receptor agonists or GLP-1 analogues, are normally prescribed for patients who have not been able to control their condition with tablet medication.

In the UK, the following incretin mimetics are available for type 2 diabetic patients - (trade name first, generic name in brackets):

- Bydureon (Exenatide) - taken once weekly
- Byetta (Exenatide) - taken twice daily

- Lyxumia (lixisenatide) - taken once daily
- Trulicity (Dulaglutide) - taken once weekly
- Victoza (Liraglutide) - taken once daily

Byetta and Bydureon are the same medical drug. The only difference is that Bydureon is long-lasting, requiring only one injection per week, whereas Byetta is taken twice-daily due to its much shorter-term effects.

They work by copying, or mimicking, the functions of the natural incretin hormones in your body that help lower post-meal blood sugar levels. These functions include:

- Stimulating the release of insulin by the pancreas after eating, even before blood sugars start to rise.
- Inhibiting the release of glucagon by the pancreas. Glucagon is a hormone that causes the liver to release its stored sugar into the bloodstream.
- Slowing glucose absorption into the bloodstream by reducing the speed at which the stomach empties after eating, thus making you feel more satisfied after a meal.

These effects are in direct response to the presence of carbohydrate in the gut and therefore the chance of significant hypoglycemia occurring is unlikely, unless used in combination with other hypoglycemic drugs.

By increasing insulin secretion and inhibiting glucagon release, incretin mimetics have blood glucose-lowering effects that help to reduce your HbA1c. They have also been shown in clinical research studies to be beneficial in losing weight, compared with a placebo, when used in combination with diet and exercise.

Now read the main points from chapter 5.

****

Main Points from Chapter 5

- For Diabetes 1, or for those with diabetes 2 who are not responding to oral medication, insulin is the only effective medication. There is only one effective way of getting it into the bloodstream, that is by injection. If it is swallowed it is only part digested and therefore its job cannot be done properly.

- Insulin is usually injected under the skin as opposed to through a vein or into a muscle. It would be injected into a vein or muscle only in special circumstances, such as if you were ill or having an operation.

- The main objective of insulin therapy is to imitate the body's natural supply as closely as possible. In a person who doesn't have diabetes, insulin is released by the pancreas in response to food. As the blood glucose levels fall between meals, so the insulin levels drop back towards zero. It never quite reaches zero and at all times there is detectable insulin in the bloodstream. What you are trying to do when you give yourself insulin injections is to reproduce the normal pattern of insulin production from the pancreas.

- For those with type 2 diabetes, there are seven different kinds of tablets and one injection treatment

Chapter 6

Advances in the Treatment of Diabetes

As can be expected, research in the treatment of diabetes is ongoing and has led to better ways of treating the condition. One such recent advance is that of the production of quick acting and longer acting insulins. Research in the UK is sponsored by both governmental organisations and also outside organisations such as pharmaceutical companies. The NHS is a major player in diabetes research

Funding research

Research that takes place in the NHS may be paid for by one of a number of different organisations, and often more than one organisation working in partnership. They include:

- the NHS, through the National Institute for Health Research (NIHR)
- the Medical Research Council (MRC)
- the Department of Health and other government departments
- medical research charities
- pharmaceutical and other healthcare companies

Through these various organisations, advances in research include:

- Development of quick acting and long acting insulins
- Better ways to monitor blood glucose and for people with diabetes to check their own blood glucose levels, including advances in non-invasive blood glucose monitoring
- Development of external insulin pumps that deliver insulin, replacing daily injections
- Successful kidney and pancreas transplantation for those whose kidneys are failing because of diabetes
- Better ways of managing diabetes in pregnant women, improving chances of successful birth
- New drugs to treat type 2 diabetes and better ways to manage it through weight control

In America, huge advances are taking place in the treatment of diabetes. Currently, scientists at the University of Texas are working on hormone therapy that could replace the need to inject insulin each day. Also, given that Diabetes is caused by the insufficient production of insulin by the pancreas. It was reported in May 2017 that the first artificial pancreas systems were beginning to infiltrate the market to help diabetics regulate their insulin levels.

To date, these are still not widely distributed, but we can expect artificial pancreas systems to become more prominent in future.

Diabetes conferences

One of the best ways to gain up-to-date knowledge of diabetes care is by attending the conferences, or getting information from www.diabetes.org.uk. The latest conference, at the time of writing was in March 2022.

Further research

One further interesting piece of research has found that Venomous sea snail venom offers fresh hope for diabetics.

The potent venom of a predatory sea snail could transform the treatment of diabetes, a 2020 study has suggested . Cone snails are found in tropical waters around the world. larger species, such as Conus geographus, which can be six inches long, release plumes of venom containing a fast-acting insulin. This causes nearby fish to experience huge falls in blood sugar, temporarily paralysing them. The snail fires a harpoon-like tooth into its prey, then pulls it into its shell to be ingested whole. Now scientists are repurposing the toxin to help people with type 1 diabetes better manage their blood sugar. Insulin, a hormone made in the pancreas, helps the body to use glucose for energy, but those with type 1 diabetes cannot produce it. Mike Lawrence, a professor of structural biology said that a faster-acting synthetic version could transform lives. "It has always been a problem with insulin injections that the body doesn't respond immediately". In a study published in *Nature Structural and Molecular Biology,* Professor Lawrence explained that human insulin contains a component that makes it clump to be stored in the pancreas. These aggregates can take an hour to break up and start working. Cone snail insulin lacks this clumping component. "We had the idea of making human insulin more snail-like", said Helena Safavi, adjunct professor of biochemistry at the University of Utah. The researchers created a version of a human insulin molecule that lacked the region responsible for clumping. Similar efforts in the past stopped the insulin working, but four components from snail insulin solved the problem. In tests with laboratory rats this hybrid molecule acted much faster than human insulin. Human trials could take place within three years.

****

Glossary of terms

Acetone: A chemical formed in the blood when the body breaks down fat instead of sugar for energy

Acidosis: Too much acid in the body, usually from the production of ketones like acetone, when cells are starved; for a person with diabetes, the most common type of acidosis is called "ketoacidosis."

Adrenal glands: Two endocrine glands that sit on top of the kidneys and make and release stress hormones, such as epinephrine (adrenaline), which stimulates carbohydrate metabolism; norepinephrine, which raises heart rate and blood pressure; and corticosteroid hormones, which control how the body utilizes fat, protein, carbohydrates, and minerals, and helps reduce inflammation.

Adult-onset diabetes: A termfor type 2 diabetes that is no longer used, because this type of diabetes is now commonly seen in children; "non-insulin dependent diabetes" is also considered an incorrect phrase in describing type 2 diabetes, because patients with this type of diabetes may at some point require insulin.

Adverse effect: Harmful effect.

Albuminuria: When kidneys become damaged, they start to leak protein in the urine. Albumin is a small, abundant protein in the blood that passes through the kidney filter into the urine easier than other proteins. Albuminuria occurs in about 30%-45% of people who have had type 1 diabetes for at least 10 years. In people newly diagnosed with type 2 diabetes, the kidneys may already show signs of small amounts of protein spillage, called "microalbuminuria."

Antibodies: Proteins that the body produces to protect itself from foreign substances, such as bacteria or viruses.

Antidiabetic agent: A substance that helps people with diabetes control the level of sugar in their blood (see insulin, oral diabetes medication).

Antigens: Substances that cause an immune response in the body, identifying substances or markers on cells; the body produces antibodies to fight antigens, or harmful substances, and tries to eliminate them.

Artery: A blood vessel that carries blood from the heart to other parts of the body; arteries are thicker than veins and have stronger, more elastic walls. Arteries sometimes develop plaque within their walls in a process known as "atherosclerosis." These plaques can become fragile and rupture, leading to complications associated with diabetes, such as heart attacks and strokes.

Artificial pancreas: A glucose sensor attached to an insulin delivery device; both are connected together by what is known as a "closed loop system." In other words, it is a system that not only can determine the body glucose level, but also takes that information and releases the appropriate amounts of insulin for the particular sugar it just measured.

Aspartame: An artificial sweetener used in place of sugar, because it has few calories; sold as "Equal" and "NutraSweet."

Asymptomatic: No symptoms; no clear sign that disease is present.

Autoimmune disease: A disorder of the body's immune system in which the immune system mistakenly attacks itself; examples of these diseases include type 1 diabetes, hyperthyroidism caused by Graves' disease, and hypothyroidism caused by Hashimoto's disease.

Autonomic neuropathy: Nerve damage to the part of the nervous system that we cannot consciously control; these nerves control our digestive system, blood vessels, urinary system, skin, and sex organs. Autonomic nerves are not under a person's control and function on their own.

Background retinopathy: This is the mildest form of eye disease caused by diabetes; it can be associated with normal vision. With a longer duration of diabetes or with uncontrolled blood sugars, eye damage can progress to more serious forms.

Basal rate: The amount of insulin required to manage normal daily blood glucose fluctuations; most people constantly produce insulin to manage the glucose fluctuations that occur during the day. In a person with diabetes, giving a constant low level amount of insulin via insulin pump mimics this normal phenomenon.

Beta cell: A type of cell in an area of the pancreas called the islets of Langerhans; beta cells make and release insulin, which helps control the glucose level in the blood.

Biosynthetic insulin: Genetically engineered human insulin; this insulin has a much lower risk of inducing an allergic reaction in people who use it, unlike cow (bovine) or pork (porcine) insulins.

Blood glucose monitoring or testing: A method of testing how much sugar is in your blood; home blood-glucose monitoring involves pricking your finger with a lancing device, putting a drop of blood on a test strip and inserting the test strip into a blood-glucose-testing meter that displays your blood glucose level. Blood-sugar testing can also be done in the laboratory.

Blood pressure: The measurement of the pressure or force of blood against the blood vessels (arteries); blood pressure is written as two numbers. The first number or top number is called the systolic pressure and is the measure of pressure in the arteries when the heart beats and pushes more blood into the arteries. The second number, called the diastolic pressure, is the pressure in the arteries when the heart rests between beats.

Brittle diabetes: When a person's blood sugar level often shifts very quickly from high to low and from low to high.

Bunion: Bump or bulge on the first joint of the big toe caused by the swelling of a sac of fluid under the skin and abnormalities in the joint; women are usually affected because of tight fitting or pointed shoes or high heels that put pressure on the toes, forcing the outward movement of the joint. People with flat feet or low arches are also prone to bunions.

Callus: A small area of skin, usually on the foot, that has become thick and hard from rubbing or pressure; calluses may lead to other problems, such as serious infection. Shoes that fit well can prevent calluses from forming.

Calorie: Energy that comes from food; some foods have more calories than others. Fats have more calories than proteins and carbohydrate. Most vegetables have few.

Carbohydrate: One of the three main classes of foods and a source of energy; carbohydrates are mainly sugars and starches that the body breaks down into glucose (a simple sugar that the body can use to feed its cells).

Cardiologist: A doctor who takes care of people with heart disease; a heart specialist.

Cardiovascular: Relating to the heart and blood vessels (arteries, veins, and capillaries).

Cholesterol: A waxy, odorless substance made by the liver that is an essential part of cell walls and nerves; cholesterol plays an important role in body functions such as digestion and hormone production.

Coma: An emergency in which a person is not conscious; may occur in people with diabetes because their blood sugar is too high or too low.

Dehydration: Large loss of body water; if a person with diabetes has a very high blood sugar level, it causes increased water loss through increased urination and therefore, extreme thirst.

Diabetic ketoacidosis (DKA): A severe, life-threatening condition that results from hyperglycemia (high blood sugar), dehydration, and acid buildup that needs emergency fluid and insulin treatment; DKA happens when there is not enough insulin and cells become starved for sugars. An alternative source of energy called ketones becomes activated. The system creates a buildup of acids. Ketoacidosis can lead to coma and even death.

Dietitian: An expert in nutrition who helps people plan the type and amount of foods to eat for special health needs; a registered dietitian (RD) has special qualifications.

Emergency medical identification: Cards, bracelets, or necklaces with a written message, used by people with diabetes or other medical problems to alert others in case of a medical emergency, such as coma.

Endocrinologist: A doctor who treats people with hormone problems.

Exchange lists: A way of grouping foods together to help people on special diets stay on the diet; each group lists food in a serving size. A person can exchange, trade, or substitute a food serving in one group for another food serving in the same group. The lists put foods into six groups: starch/bread, meat, vegetables, fruit, milk, and fats. Within a food group, one serving of each food item in that group has about the same amount of carbohydrate, protein, fat, and calories.

Fats: Substances that help the body use some vitamins and keep the skin healthy; they are also the main way the body stores energy. In food, there are many types of fats -- saturated, unsaturated, polyunsaturated, monounsaturated, and trans fats.

Fructose: A type of sugar found in many fruits and vegetables and in honey; fructose is used to sweeten some diet foods, but this type of sweetener is typically not recommended for people with diabetes, because it could have a negative effect on blood sugar.

Gangrene: The death of body tissues, usually due to a lack of blood supply, especially in the legs and feet.

Gastroparesis: A form of nerve damage that affects the stomach and intestines; with this condition, food is not digested properly and does not move through the stomach and intestinal tract normally. It can result in nausea and vomiting, because the transit time of food is slowed by nerve damage.

Gestational diabetes: A high blood sugar level that starts or is first recognized during pregnancy; hormone changes during pregnancy affect the action of insulin, resulting in high blood sugar levels. Usually, blood sugar levels return to normal after childbirth.

Glaucoma: An eye disease associated with increased pressure within the eye; glaucoma can damage the optic nerve and cause impaired vision and blindness.

Glucose: A simple sugar found in the blood; it is the body's main source of energy; also known as "dextrose."

Glucose tolerance test: A test to determine if a person has diabetes; the test is done in a lab or doctor's office in the morning before the person has eaten. A period of at least 8 hours without any food is recommended prior to doing the test.

High blood pressure: A condition when the blood flows through the blood vessels at a force greater than normal; high blood pressure strains the heart, harms the arteries, and increases the risk of heart attack, stroke, and kidney problems; also called "hypertension."

Home blood glucose monitoring: A way in which a person can test how much sugar is in the blood; also called "self-monitoring of blood glucose

Hormone: A chemical released in one organ or part of the body that travels through the blood to another area, where it helps to control certain bodily functions; for instance, insulin is a hormone made by the beta cells in the pancreas and when released, it triggers other cells to use glucose for energy.

Human insulin: Bio-engineered insulin very similar to insulin made by the body; the DNA code for making human insulin is put into bacteria or yeast cells and the insulin made is purified and sold as human insulin.

Hyperglycemia: High blood sugar; this condition is fairly common in people with diabetes. Many things can cause hyperglycemia. It occurs when the body does not have enough insulin or cannot use the insulin it does have.

Hypoglycemia: Low blood sugar; the condition often occurs in people with diabetes. Most cases occur when there is too much insulin and not enough glucose in your body.

Injection sites: Places on the body where people can inject insulin most easily.

Insulin: A hormone produced by the pancreas that helps the body use sugar for energy; the beta cells of the pancreas make insulin.

Insulin mixture: A mixture of insulin that contains short-, intermediate- or long-acting insulin; you can buy premixed insulin to eliminate the need for mixing insulin from two bottles.

Insulin pump: A small, computerized device that is worn on a belt or put in a pocket; insulin pumps have a small flexible tube with a fine needle on the end. The needle is inserted under the skin of the abdomen and taped in place. A carefully measured, steady flow of insulin is released into the body.

Insulin reaction: Another term for hypoglycemia in a person with diabetes; this occurs when a person with diabetes has injected too much insulin, eaten too little food, or has exercised without eating extra food.

Insulin receptors: Areas on the outer part of a cell that allow insulin in the blood to join or bind with the cell; when the cell and insulin bind together, the cell can take glucose from the blood and use it for energy.

Insulin resistance: When the effect of insulin on muscle, fat, and liver cells becomes less effective; this effect occurs with both insulin produced in the body and with insulin injections. Therefore, higher levels of insulin are needed to lower the blood sugar.

Lancet: A fine, sharp pointed needle for pricking the skin; used in blood sugar monitoring.

Laser treatment: The use of a strong beam of light (laser) to heal a damaged area; a person with diabetes might receive laser treatments to heal blood vessels in the eye.

Late-onset diabetes: Former term used for type 2 diabetes.

Lipid: Another term for a fat or fat-like substance in the blood; the body stores fat as energy for future use, just like a car that has a reserve fuel tank.

Metabolism: All of the physical and chemical processes in the body that occur when food is broken down, energy is created and wastes are produced.

Mg/dL (milligrams per deciliter): Measurement that indicates the amount of a particular substance such as glucose in a specific amount of blood.

Mixed dose: A prescribed dose of insulin in which two types of insulin are combined and injected at once; a mixed dose commonly combines a fast-acting and longer-acting insulin. A mixed dose can either come in a pre-mixed syringe or mixed at the time of injection. A mixed dose may be prescribed to provide better blood sugar control.

Nephropathy: Disease of the kidneys caused by damage to the small blood vessels or to the units in the kidneys that clean the blood; people who have had diabetes for a long time may develop nephropathy.

Neurologist: A doctor who treats people who have problems of the nervous system (brain, spinal cord, and nerves).

Neuropathy: Nerve damage; people who have had diabetes that is not well controlled may develop nerve damage.

Non-insulin dependent diabetes: Former term for type 2 diabetes.

Obesity: A term uses to describe excess body fat; it is defined in terms of a person's weight and height, or his/her body mass index (BMI). A BMI over 30 is classified as being obese. Obesity makes your body less sensitive to insulin's action. Extra body fat is thought to be a risk factor for diabetes.

Ophthalmologist: A doctor who treats people with eye diseases.

Optometrist: A person professionally trained to test the eyes and to detect and treat eye problems, as well as some diseases, by prescribing and adapting corrective lenses.

Oral diabetes medications: Medications that people take to lower the level of sugar in the blood; oral diabetes medications are prescribed for people whose pancreas still produces some insulin.

Pancreas-a large gland behind the stomach-produced a substance that regulated the level of blood glucose, stopped it rising.

Peak action: The time when the effect of something is as strong as it can be, such as when insulin is having the most effect on blood sugar.

Periodontal disease: Damage to the gums and tissues around the teeth; people who have diabetes are more likely to have periodontal disease than people who do not have diabetes.

Peripheral neuropathy: A type of nerve damage most commonly affecting the feet and legs.

Podiatrist: A health professional who diagnoses and treats foot problems.

Polydipsia: Excessive thirst that lasts for long periods of time; may be a sign of diabetes.

Polyphagia: Excessive hunger and eating; may be a sign of diabetes.

Polyunsaturated fat: A type of fat that can be substituted for saturated fats in the diet and can reduce LDL "bad" cholesterol.

Polyuria: Increased need to urinate often; a common sign of diabetes.

Protein: One of three main classes of food; proteins are made of amino acids, which are called the "building blocks of the cells."

Rapid-acting Insulin: Covers insulin needs for meals eaten at the same time as the injection; this type of insulin is used with longer-acting insulin. Includes Humalog, Novolog, and Apidra.

Regular insulin: A type of insulin that is rapid-acting.

Renal: Relating to the kidneys.

Retina: The center part of the back lining of the eye that senses light; it has many small blood vessels that are sometimes harmed when a person has had diabetes for a long time.

Retinopathy: A disease of the small blood vessels in the retina of the eye.

Risk factor: Anything that increases the chance of a person developing a disease or condition.

Saccharin: An artificial sweetener that is used in place of sugar because it has no calories and does not increase blood sugar.

Self-blood glucose monitoring: See home blood glucose monitoring.

Short-acting Insulin: Covers insulin needs for meals eaten within 30-60 minutes; includes humulin or novolin, or Velosulin (in an insulin pump).

Sucrose: Table sugar; a form of sugar that the body must break down into a more simple form before the blood can absorb it and take it to the cells.

Sucralose: An artificial sweetener that is 600 times sweeter than sugar; can be used in cooking. Splenda is a brand name of sucralose.

Sugar: A class of carbohydrates that tastes sweet; sugar is a quick and easy fuel for the body to use. Some types of sugar are lactose, glucose, fructose, and sucrose.

Sulfonylureas: Pills or capsules that people take to lower the level of sugar in the blood; these oral diabetic medications work to lower your blood sugar by making your pancreas produce more insulin.

Triglyceride: Fats carried in the blood from the food we eat; most of the fats we eat, including butter, margarines, and oils, are in triglyceride form. Excess triglycerides are stored in fat cells throughout the body. The body needs insulin to remove this type of fat from the blood.

Type 1 diabetes: A type of diabetes in which the insulin-producing cells (called beta cells) of the pancreas are damaged; people with type 1 diabetes produce little or no insulin, so glucose cannot get into the body's cells for use as energy. This causes blood sugar to rise. People with type 1 diabetes must use insulin injections to control their blood sugar.

Type 2 diabetes: A type of diabetes in which the insulin produced is either not enough or the person's body does not respond normally to the amount present; therefore, glucose in the blood cannot get into the body's cells for use as energy. This results in an increase in the level of glucose (sugar) in the blood.

Ulcer: A break in the skin; a deep sore. People with diabetes may develop ulcers from minor scrapes on the feet or legs, from cuts that heal slowly, or from the rubbing of shoes that don't fit well. Ulcers can become infected and should be treated promptly.

Unit of insulin: The basic measure of insulin; U-100 is the most common concentration of insulin. U-100 means that there are 100 units of insulin per milliliter (ml) of liquid. For the occasional patient who has severe insulin resistance, insulin is available as a U-500 form.

Urine testing: Checking urine to see if it contains ketones; if you have type 1 diabetes, are pregnant and have diabetes, or have gestational diabetes, your doctor may ask you to check your urine for ketones. This is an easy test done at home with a dipstick measure.

Urologist: A doctor who specializes in treatment of the urinary tract for men and women, as well as treatment of the genital organs for males.

Vaginitis: An inflammation or infection of the vaginal tissues; a woman with this condition may have itching or burning or vaginal discharge. Women who have diabetes may develop vaginitis more often than women who do not have diabetes.

Vein: A blood vessel that carries blood to the heart.

Vitrectomy: A procedure in which the gel from the center of the eyeball is removed because it has blood and scar tissue that blocks vision; an eye surgeon replaces the clouded gel with a clear fluid.

Xylitol: A nutritive sweetener used in dietary foods; it is a sugar alcohol that the body uses slowly, and contains fewer calories than table sugar.

****

Useful Addresses and Websites

Age UK

Travis House,

1-6 Travis Square

London

WC1H 9NA

Advice line; 0800 055 6112

Website; www.ageuk.org.uk

Benefit Enquiry Line / Disability Benefits

Website: www.gov.uk/disability-benefits-helpline

Blood Pressure Association

Wolfson Institute of Preventative Medicine

Charterhouse square

London EC1M 6BQ

Information line; 020 7882 6218

Website: www.bloodpressureuk.org

Carers UK

20 Great Dover Street

London SE1 4LX

Helpline: 0808 808 7777

Website; www.carersuk.org

Carers Wales

Unit 5

Ynys Bridge Court

Cardiff CF15 9SS

t: 029 2081 1370

Carers Scotland

The Cottage

21 Pearce Street

Glasgow G51 3UT

t: 0141 445 3070

Carers Northern Ireland

58 Howard Street

Belfast BT1 6JP

t: 02890 439 843

Department of Health and Social Care

Richmond House

39 Victoria Street

London SW1H OEU

Website: www.gov.uk

Diabetes UK

Wells Lawrence House

126 Back Church Lane

London

E1 1FH

Tel: 0345 123 2399 (Mon-Fri, 9am-7pm)

Website: www.diabetes.org.uk

Disabled Living Foundation

Email: info@dlf.org.uk

Helpline: 0300 999 0004 (Mom- Fri 10am-4pm)

Website: www.dlf.org.uk

DVA (Driver and Vehicle Licensing Agency)

DVLA

Swansea SA6 7JL

www.gov.uk/government/organisations/driver-and-vehice-licensing-agency

Disabled Motoring UK

Headquarters, Ashwelthorpe

Norwich NR16 1EX

Tel: 01508 489449

Website: www.disableddmotoring.org

National Institute for Health and Care Excellence

(NICE) (London office)

2nd Floor, 2 Redman Place

London E20 1JQ

Tel: 0300 323 0140

Website: www.nice.org.uk

NHS 111

Tel: 111 (24 hours, 365 days a year)

Website: www.nhs.uk/nhsengland

NHS England

Te: 0300 311 2233 (Mon-Fri 8am-6pm)

Website: www.england.nhs.uk

Health and Social Care in Northern Ireland

Website: www.hscni.net

NHS Scotland

Website: www.show.scot.nhs.uk

NHS Direct Wales

Tel: 0845 4647

Website: www.nhsdirect.wales.nhs.uk

Royal National Institute of Blind People (RNIB)

Tel: 0303 123 9999

Website: www.rnib.org.uk

Weight Watchers

Website: www.weightwatchers.com

Healthtalk

Website: www.healthtalk.org

NHS choices

Website: www.nhs.uk/conditions

Patient UK

Website: www.patient.info

Runsweet.com

Website: www.runsweet.com

For people with Type 1 Diabetes

****

Index

Metformin SR (slow release, 115
Mild hypos, 46
Monitoring glucose, 4, 49
Muscle movement, 84, 106

National Institute for Health Research (NIHR), 127
Natural remedies, 5, 96
Nausea, 34, 47, 104
Nephropathy, 142
Nerve Damage, 65
NHS, 85, 121, 127, 152, 153

Obesity, 143
Okra, 97, 104
Omega-3, 92
Oral medication, 5, 86, 107, 125
Oriental medicine, 97

Pancreas, 21, 144
Parents, 25
Pioglitazone (Actos, 117
Plant-based therapies, 97
Podiatrist, 144
Podiatry, 70
Polyglandular autoimmune syndrome, 26
Polyuria, 23
Potatoes, 90
Prandial glucose regulators, 44, 118, 119
Pregnant women, 11
Preventing hypoglycemia, 4, 46
Processed foods, 94
Protein, 22, 92, 93, 95, 131, 132, 137
Pulses, 5, 91, 92
Rapid lateral flow, 8
Red blood cells, 92

****

Further titles in the Emerald Explaining Series

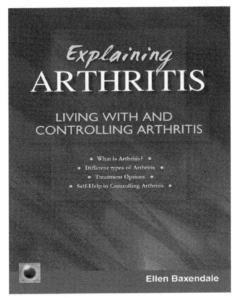

ISBN 978-1-84716-967-9 £9.99

Everyone has heard of arthritis and knows someone with the condition. However, if we ourselves are not affected by the condition we tend not to know much about it. Arthritis is a common condition that causes joint inflammation and pain, and it affects about 10 million people in the UK. People of all ages can get it and there are many forms of the condition such as Osteo-arthritis, Rheumatoid Arthritis and Gout.

This book will provide you with the information you need to understand this condition in all its different forms, the treatment options available to you, different methods of coping, and where to go for further advice and help. It will also, importantly, help you see the 'wood from the trees' and avoid the many offers of treatment in the form of pills and potions that seek to exploit the sufferer.

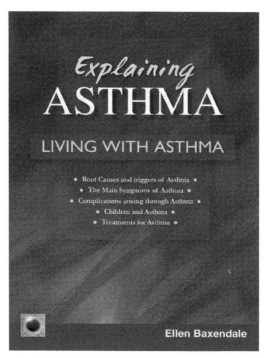

978-184716-966-2   £9.99

Asthma is a common lung condition that causes breathing difficulties. with varying degrees of severity. It affects people of all ages and often starts in childhood, although it can also develop for the first time in adults. There's currently no cure, but there are simple treatments that can help keep the symptoms under control so it doesn't have a big impact on your life.

This comprehensive book looks at the causes of asthma and what can be done to alleviate them and what treatments are available. The book also looks at the things that can be done by the individual to minimise the effects of asthma.

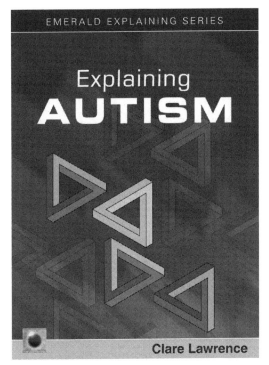

EMERALD EXPLAINING SERIES

Explaining
AUTISM

Clare Lawrence

978-1-84716-726-2 £9.99

What is autism? With perhaps one in a hundred of our population now receiving a diagnosis of Autism, this is a question that more and more people are asking.

'Explaining Autism is the Second Edition of this highly successful book in the 'Explaining' series and provides a clear and concise introduction to this fascinating and perplexing subject. Written in accessible, non-specialist language it provides an ideal introduction for parents, carers, teachers and employers – for anyone coming across this intriguing condition – on ways to understand what is Autism

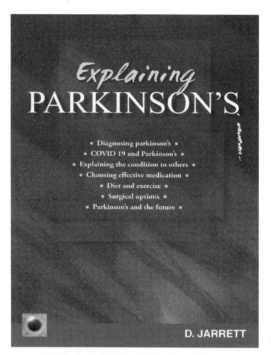

978-1-84716-660-9 £9.99

Parkinson's, or the onset of Parkinson's, is a very stressful time for those unfortunate to suffer it. Quite often guidance on the subject is conflicting and unclear.

This Third Edition of *Explaining Parkinson's* deals with Parkinson's in a very sensitive and clear way and will be of great assistance and comfort to those who read it. The book gives advice on techniques for coping with the diagnosis, finding the right doctors, diets and, overall, dealing with the condition and the attendant stress.